Endorsements for *Admissions*

This cacophony of own voice narratives broadens the conversation around mental health in Australia.

Maxine Beneba Clarke

Admissions moved me to tears. It is an anthology both connected and disconnected, an echo of the mental illness and recovery, the isolation and community experienced by the authors. With fearlessness, anger and gracious vulnerability, this collection bleeds and heals and bleeds again. Each piece is extremely special, and extremely important: a howl into the void, a loving ode to selves, and a bearing witness. We are lucky to have these writers, and these words.

Laura Helen McPhee-Browne

Significant and compelling.

Claudia Karvan

T0363110

Edited by David Stavanger,
Radhiah Chowdhury and
Mohammad Awad

Admissions

UPSWELL

First published in Australia in 2022
by Upswell Publishing
Perth, Western Australia
upswellpublishing.com

ISBN: 978-0-6452480-9-8

 A catalogue record for this
book is available from the
National Library of Australia

Cover design by Chil3, Fremantle
Typeset in Foundry Origin by Lasertype
Printed by McPherson's Printing Group

with_ architecture
studio

With_ Architectural Studio in Perth has generously enabled Sam Gorecki,
their Creative Lead (Graphics), to design the cover of this book for Upswell
using the commissioned artwork of Amani Haydar. This support is a fine
demonstration of an integral interest in cultural work driving generosity
and solidarity from a private business.

Index

Introduction

Mental health has never enjoyed such prevalence in the national conversation nor such generosity of funding outbursts than in recent times, fuelled in the main by the impact of a pandemic and the proliferation of public health platforms and initiatives encouraging us all to talk openly about whether we're okay or some shade of blue. Even urinals have posters at eye level to remind us that men feel things, too.

While this amplified discourse is great, broadening and foregrounding mental health as something we all go through in an attempt to destigmatise (even legitimise), for many of us with lived experience of chronic mental illness, acute florid episodes and truly labile states, not to mention those who are ongoing consumers – often consumed by mental health as a private and public institution – there is an underlying sense of being more alone, unseen and very much unheard in the bureaucratic narrative of *we're all in this together*. There has also been a loss of degree, nuance and the larger spectrum of experience within psychiatric labels. Then there are the other factors inherent to poor and deteriorating mental health that no one in power wants to touch with a blank cheque, that no prescription can fill, and that no GP-signed care plan can overcome, not the least of which are a far-from-robust Eurocentric view of diagnosis, treatment and illness, alongside the ravages of loneliness, costs of living and capitalism. Most people within this system need the solid and secure foundation of a home, food and real connection to community ahead of a free morning tea with a random well-intended stranger in a branded t-shirt telling us that a conversation can change a life (maybe it can, but it can't pay rent or be cashed at Woolworths).

Across the entire span of this collection of 105 voices within mental health, the DSM is surprisingly mentioned only twice (once highlighting that a dislike of peas is strangely not yet a diagnostic criteria). The Diagnostic and Statistical Manual of Mental Disorders (the DSM, now up to its fifth sequel, equal to both the Die Hard franchise and the Twilight saga, but with more enduring merch) is the clinical bible that mental health professionals turn to to classify (and attempt to communicate) a patient's diagnosis. The whole mental health machine is founded on it, from initial assessments that can reshape a life in less than an hour to psychiatric opinion based on (pseudo)science, to public health assessments defining individual rights, to insurance companies using the coding system to decide who gets reimbursed for care, to good old Big Pharmaceutical reframing criteria to repurpose drugs with expired patents for ever-increasing profit.

We want to be upfront about something: this anthology is not based on labelling people or pathologising psychological distress as a spectator sport. We haven't categorised this collection that way nor asked anyone to identify via diagnosis. Its position is not anti-psychiatry, though no psychiatrists were consulted or commissioned; none of the editors have financial ties or association with Big Pharma, though we are all open advocates of Big Poetry. Many people within these pages are on or recovering from scripted drugs, a baseline fact with some noted benefits and a wide range of side effects. This has not been forged as the antithesis of the DSM and its ilk, as that reduces the true value and hard-won insights held in these varied lives and lines.

To be clearer, here are five ways this anthology is not like the DSM-5:

- The selection of these pieces was not based on the medicalisation of human nature

- It doesn't discount the cultural, gendered and ethnic diversity and experiences of individuals

- This is a reliable (non)standardised poetic take on mental health in all its forms

- It celebrates (un)common language and upends the standard criteria of madness

- Everything within these pages is someone's truth

There is no way to neatly summarise what *Admissions* is or what it contains. If we were to write shorthand case notes to hand it over to you as a reader, they would say:

Dolphins. Cicada shells. Frozen lakes. Armpits. Dettol lakes. Clinical Depression. Trauma. Colonialism. Ambulances. Beethoven. Kanye. King prawns. I-phones. Driftwood. Invisibility. Capitalism. Sore Hearts. Body dysmorphia. Body dysphoria. Dr Dre. Tia Kofi. Ally McBeal. Tori Amos. Princess Diana. Glee. Carl Jung. Carl Sagan. David Bowie. David Byrne. Hospitalisation. Isolation. Covid. Consent. Anxiety. Loss of Agency. Delusions. Dissociation. Smart Ovens. Discount Supermen. St John's Wort. Angels. Tumblr. Tupperware. The Tardis. Domestic violence. Institutionalisation. Racism. Eating Disorders. ECT. OCD. Californian bungalows. Psychologists' floors. Playing dress-up. Surgical gowns. Buzzed heads. Precious metals. Bill Gates. Bi cats. Hissing Apples. Sexual Assault. Acute Distress. Covid. Prolonged. Homelessness. Poverty. PTSD. Blue ladies. Glad Wrap. Glass pipes. Fibulas. Freud's couch. Fat Yaks. Ancestors. Ramadan. Prayers. Grief. Coercive practice. Seclusion. Autism. Suicide. Psychosis. Schizophrenia. Schizoaffective. Devil's Ivy. Sundresses. Pineapple pizza. Snails. Magicians. Super-eights. WestConnex. Uno. Addiction. Twelve steps. ADHD. Insomnia. Incarceration. Mania. Memories. Exploitation. Boree Creek. The Gap. Lego. Feathers. Lithium. The secret paths of possums. Cursory Google searches. Bullying. Rage. Elegy. Millennial condition. Visiting hours. Metamorphosis. Bad medicine. Calling In. Dogs. Wolves. So many canines. Too many Zooms. So many flipped moons.

None of this is word salad. None of this needs to be dressed up in the language suit of clinicians.

This anthology initially grew out of a movement that has been gaining momentum at the fringes of an often-narrow media discourse. The term *lived experience* in a mental ill-health context can refer to either a consumer, carer or both: someone who has actually gone through it. In this anthology, we have actively chosen to foreground the voices of those who have directly experienced mental health issues themselves, with a strong emphasis throughout of work that amplifies many who have been (and still are) part of the public health system in this country. This anthology walks in the steps made by the established international MAD Pride movement and the growing MAD Poetry community (which proudly originated in the Illawarra region), both of which formed to reclaim demeaning institutional language/ descriptors and to present the diverse phenomena of 'madness' as sources of identity, culture, possibility and, in this case, life-affirming poetry and prose. We want to acknowledge all the contributors here with a lived experience of mental ill-health and recovery (and the experience of people who have been carers, families or supporters), and any readers and the thousands of people who also deserve to have their voices amplified in print. In particular, we want to acknowledge the First Nations writers who kindly agreed to have their work included, and the ongoing lateral violence, intergenerational trauma and dispossession they encounter in many mental health settings and across our broader society. Always was, always will be Aboriginal land.

Our intention as editors of this collection is to eschew gatekeeping wherever possible, and opt instead for radical empathy, inclusivity and generosity. To that end, this collection accommodates not only familiar, 'established' contributors (although whose establishment are we talking about here?), but also a spectacular cohort of new voices gathered via a general call-out with Red Room Poetry. Would that we had the scope to include all the submissions that came through that call-out, for each one brought its own generously offered truth and experienced reality. Faced with the prosaic tyrannies of page extent and word count, however, we have sought in our selection to represent as wide and diverse a range of mental health experiences and poetic forms as possible. The twin dragons of racism and colonialism extend to all our contributors from the global majority, whose writing is inevitably informed by the oft-violent harvests at the intersections of displacement, minorisation and mental health. While it is certainly true that mental illness is resoundingly democratic in its reach, its experience and effects both within and without traditional Western frameworks is undoubtedly impacted by considerations of the historical and cultural contexts of race, class, gender, ability and all the other granular ways we can experience trauma and exclusion.

Before this collection became *Admissions*, one of our editorial triumvirate, Mohammad Awad, was running twelve-week poetry therapy groups across various mental health wards in New South Wales as a peer worker. Poetry occupying the environs of psychiatrists and psychologists, with poets as the new practitioners on the psych ward (yet we've always been here, mostly involuntarily). *North and South* became symbols of bipolar, imagery of scattered jigsaw pieces reflected a diagnosis's capacity for destruction of the self, *A thousand and one voices* an allegory for psychosis, all coexisting in an environment where labels are routinely thrust upon patients. Having a facilitator with lived experience aided in destigmatising mental illness, while providing participants with the language to articulate their inner worlds and celebrate the artistry they possessed, leading people to share their poetry in all spaces, from clinical sessions to mental health review tribunals. The 'mad person' no longer mocked for reciting poetry in the hospital halls.

There is a tendency within popular culture to fetishise both mental illness and trauma, as though 'good art' cannot be created without pain, as though 'resilience' is the marker of 'good artists' (and, conversely, that if we cannot be 'resilient' and 'brave', we are somehow less admirable or convincing as artists and human beings), as though adversity is to be desired and even sought out when embarking on artistic work. *Admissions* is not intended as a work of trauma porn or voyeurism where art is fed by suffering. We are rather guided by the ways in which art and language can expiate suffering. Art as release, art as relief, art as recovery, remission, remediation. Group therapy on an individual and community scale. We are profoundly indebted to the bountiful generosity of all those who have contributed to this collective expiation with their excoriating rage, heart-wrenching grief, gut-busting humour and deep, abiding humanity, and also to the several artists who initially agreed to join this collection and subsequently withdrew as their own mental health journeys suffered setbacks due to the myriad pressures of existing ethically in our current reality.

Within these pages is a cohort of activist consumers, neurodivergent creatives, psychiatric and trauma survivors, fringe dreamers, community leaders and mind-bending writers. It is the lived experience within these pages (including the three of us as editors) that shapes this collection. We are the collective architects of this anthology, the creators of poetry as a new prototype of how language can be constructed in this space not to censor or constrain, but as an act of sovereignty, self-care and self-determination.

David, Radhiah and Mohammad

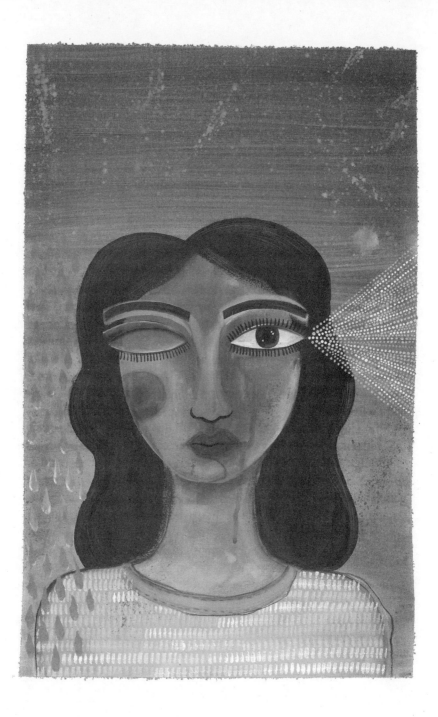

We're painting our faces and dressing in thoughts from the skies

David Bowie, 'After All', 1970

who is she

Manal Younus

who is she
the one who shares your face
but not your vision

sliced between selves
one of joy
while the other delves
into desolation
a place of your own creation

when your body is worn
hers is worn out
your heart torn
hers
torn out

it is easier to believe she does not exist
than to reach into the abyss
only to find your own reflection
the true victim of your deception

you smother her
to claim heroism
but perhaps
to save one's self
is the most heroic act

for without her,
who are you?
– my

No crazy person is mad enough

Fiona Wright

My girlfriend and I were outed on our very first date. On both of them – by which I mean on both the date that I've always considered our first, where we met for coffee on a weekend morning and could easily have talked all day, and also on the date a few days later, from which she begins her tally. Before that, she always says, neither of us knew that we were interested. And, therefore, the coffee doesn't count. But I have never been a fan of ambiguity and so place my beginning at the very beginning – it's more clear-cut that way.

On that first date, at the very beginning, I arrived early. I always do this when I'm meeting people who I don't know well because I know there is little chance that I will recognise them. I can't remember faces; I learned instead, without even realising that I was doing it, to rely on other details – hairstyle or mannerisms or gait or shape or stance or smell – to distinguish between people and identify my loved ones. It works well with friends and family (mostly – I once introduced myself to my best and oldest friend at his own front door because he'd grown a truly impressive beard since I'd last seen him). It works less well with casual acquaintances, though; and it does not work at all with relative strangers. Arriving early, sitting somewhere prominent, and taking out a book – this means the onus is on the other person to find and recognise me. They do this so easily and unthinkingly, most of the time, that the skill of it isn't something they notice.

So at the very beginning, I was there early. She was late. She always is, I know this now, and she apologised, breathlessly, as she swept in.

You look like you've been here a while, she said, contrite. I smiled and said I'd been perfectly happy reading away, and added that my over-punctuality was done on purpose.

I'm faceblind, I said, so I—

Faceblind? she cut me off, confused. It's a reaction I am used to given how few people have ever heard of the condition, so much so that I have an explanation I recite almost by rote. I say its medical name (prosopagnosia) because that seems to lend it some validity, I say that I can indeed see faces, just not remember them, that sometimes, yes, I am thrown by my own— but this too she interrupted.

You can't be faceblind, she said, and the bluntness of the assertion I did not know how to take. It took a few more very confused exchanges until we both realised what the other meant. She'd been startled by my declaration because she too is prosopagnostic – and meeting another person who shared this way of being in the world was the last thing that she had expected from that morning.

We could easily have talked all day. We talked about all kinds of things – art and data and neuroscience and books and jobs and mythology – and we also talked about our most embarrassing moments of misrecognition (I once mistook a stranger's toddler for my niece, she once told Tilda Swinton how much she loved Tilda Swinton), all the little tactics we employ when we have no idea with whom it is that we are talking, though they clearly know us quite well. For the record: I ask question after question after question, probing for a detail that might help me figure it out – and the moment that the penny drops I look away because I know the realisation clearly dawns across my face.

On our first date, at the later, less absolute beginning (the beginning she insists upon), my girlfriend and I met in the outside bar of a shabby theatre. We had swapped selfies while we were both in transit because I'd realised, with some horror, that I'd had my hair cut a few days before and had most likely thereby rendered my face unrecognisable to her; I was unconvinced that I'd be able to identify hers within a crowd. I found her by her outfit: the hot-pink shirt that was in frame in the photo she had sent.

We had only just found each other, just started talking, when a tall, elfin-faced woman came up beside us, waving with both hands despite the sweating beer held in the left. She was beaming with all her might, so I smiled back and said hello. She launched into all the usual small-talk questions, and my girlfriend's responses were warm and funny and full of cheer. I nodded along, laughed in the right places, answered the questions deliberately directed my way in an effort to include me in the conversation. And how's your work going? my girlfriend asked, and the woman laughed it off, and changed the subject briefly before beginning to wander back to her friends. It's lovely to see you both, she added, tossing her pale hair.

Who was that? I asked my girlfriend.

I thought you knew her? she replied, eyes wide.

She's not your friend?

I don't know, maybe?

I don't think—

A half-smile and an eyebrow askew. What passed between us then was a quiet, wondrous disbelief that both of us were experiencing this same ridiculously absurd thing, and without the usual dissonance of knowing it is not shared. I looked away first. The theatre bell rang. And it was only after we moved inside, into the murmuring half-dark, that it hit me.

Oh god, I said, before I even knew that I was speaking. Our friend—

You got it? You know her?

Her work – she said something about being a nurse?

Yes, she— my girlfriend paused. Oh god. Her voice almost a groan.

My nurse, I said, and it was both a statement and a question.

Mine too.

Yeah.

She flicked her thumb against the fingers of her right hand a few times, quickly. I couldn't read her face.

So psych wards, I said, with a too-bright levity I hoped might defuse the tension. Part of both of our lives?

She laughed then, and it was a full-throated, beautiful thing.

My girlfriend and I still joke about this, being outed on that date – we would have discovered this shared detail on our own soon enough, especially because neither of us sets any store by secrecy as far as illness is concerned. The story is one we love to tell, and it is so often met with that squeamish, cringey kind of horror that witnessing acute embarrassment or shame evokes. But even at the time we weren't ashamed; and while it felt awkward to have had the moment of disclosure chosen for us, the relief, for both of us, was palpable. If anything, we had been spared a conversation we would otherwise have overburdened. And more than anything else, we found the whole thing hilarious. We still do.

Later that night we determined that we had always been at different locations of the same hospital chain, and always at different times. But because our mutual acquaintance worked in all its locations, and had met so many people right across them, she had assumed she'd met us simultaneously, that we had been on a ward together, and knew each other because of that.

The performance started, and my girlfriend started shifting her weight rhythmically in her chair, backward and forward, her thumb still flicking. She saw me looking, turned her face towards mine without quite meeting it. She said, by the way, I sometimes—

I get it, I said, and I will never forget the way she smiled.

At the hospital we'd both stayed in at different times, relationships between patients were explicitly forbidden. This is common practice, and the reasons given vary: it's because of safety, privacy, emotional vulnerability, it's because sex might be symptomatic, or the capacity to consent complicated, it's because the relationship might interfere with treatment, or each illness exacerbate the other. I mention this only because I remember laughing when the intake nurse first explained this rule to me. I remember saying, surely no crazy person is mad enough to want to date another crazy person. Surely. She was, of course, unimpressed.

It was bombast, even now my most instinctual response to nervousness or fear. And my bombast was defensive, a weapon really aimed directly back at me. Because surely, I believed, surely no one could be mad enough to want to spend their time or share their life with me. Especially because that would inevitably mean spending time with my illness as well, and any sane person would find that whole situation intolerable.

When the fact of my girlfriend's illness first came up in conversation with my family – one of those early conversations, where I was still shy and they still demonstrably careful – there was a momentary and entirely unintended exhalation, clearly audible. I'm not sure whose breath it was that caught that way, could tell that it was instantly regretted, all the more so when we all left it unacknowledged, as if ignoring it could mean it hadn't happened. After a small pause, my mother said kindly, I guess you can look after each other?

Yes, I replied. And I thought, isn't that supposed to always be the way?

My girlfriend was hospitalised again somewhere around six months after that strange and wonderful night at the theatre, more as a pre-emptive move than out of acute distress. I visited as soon as I was able, driving north, instead of west, along the quiet, curling bays on the other side of the harbour, the streets overarched with thick-barked trees, the air chittering with cicadas. I was taken aback by how similar the building seemed despite its water views – the same layout, the same carpet, the same frosted glass partitions; I perched on the end of the bed (the same waffle-weave cotton blanket) and watched her unpack her clothes into the little laminex wardrobe beside the door. A nurse knocked then tucked his head around the doorframe, quietly reminding her to go downstairs for dinner, and then he left – and left me gobsmacked for the gentleness of his appeal.

When we did walk down those stairs a little later – a single flight with a sudden kink in the middle, just like in my hospital – we stepped into the dining room, and I froze. I didn't want to, nor mean to; I kept thinking, this cannot be about you, it cannot, not now. I forced myself to move, to walk alongside her, I gathered her cutlery and some little sachets of mayonnaise. The basket, with its obsessively tidy line of single-serve condiments, was exactly the same. The flimsy-looking fruit bowl was exactly the same. The juice dispenser and the coffee machine, the conveyor-belt toaster, the cross-hatched non-slip mats beneath them all, the same. The stack of plastic trays at the counter were the same, and behind the counter the bain-maries held a meal that was the same – a Keen's powder curry with halved hard-boiled eggs staring up out of the sauce – and I could almost taste it in my throat just from the smell. This cannot be about you, not right now.

We were late enough that no one else was in the room, that a purplish light from the setting sun was splayed across the carpet where we sat at the table by the window. A gang of lorikeets began to shriek and giggle in the garden's native fig. The first time she'd come here, she said, the lorikeets seemed like a miracle: she grew up overseas, and in this country has only lived within the urban centre of the city. We were quiet. I could barely think. She lay her hand over mine, balled up there on the table, and she looked at me, a question.

The dining room is just the same, I said, and she nodded, and I knew I didn't have to explain.

I don't think I realised, at the beginning, how important this is, how much difference it makes. To not have to explain, to never have to step through all those intricate, contradictory and tangled emotions and ideas, the old hurts and odd fears and the forceful bodily reactions, everything that tramples through us when our minds are at their most unruly. How much difference it makes to not have to explain each thing that makes me different, and thereby be reminded of that difference every time, but instead to have something of it understood or even shared. We don't point out or try to refute the illogic of the other's illness. We do not offer platitudes, or any of those well-meaning consolations or suggestions (It will get better! Stay positive! You should try yoga!) when the other is struggling or in pain. We don't force each other and don't lay blame. But what is most important is that we both know, intimately and all too well, that most of the time there's nothing anyone can do, no solution or salve that might be found. And so all we do is stay. We just stay there, sometimes talking, sometimes silent, but certainly, solidly there.

That this is what it means to share a way of being in the world I had no way of knowing. I did not even recognise the lack.

For a long time, I would flush with a thick, hot grief whenever I thought of all the pain that had radiated outwards from the epicentre of my illness, all the people who love me and had absorbed it. All that worry and all that fear, all that helplessness and horror, pity and confusion and anger and loss: I felt wretched for everything I'd put them through. That's how I always phrased it – in the active voice, with me the agent, the cause. That's how I phrased it, even when I was trying so hard to remember, in the hope that I might eventually believe, that my illness wasn't something I had brought upon myself. It took much longer to understand that it wasn't me who had so hurt the people around me than it did to accept that I couldn't have prevented my illness, that nothing I did or could have done would have made any difference at all. In part, this latter was made easier by new research and diagnostic models that are beginning to understand things like genetic predisposition, brain structure and processing, minority stress – all of which seem tangible to me, more or less, and far beyond a person's remit or control. But it is only now, standing on this other side of that equation, where I am caring as well as being cared for, that the former is starting to shift.

Because living with another person's illness isn't easy, but it's not as hard as I'd imagined. It hurts sometimes, but not as much as I had thought it must, and certainly far less intensely than experiencing the illness firsthand. Sometimes it's frustrating and repetitive and tiring – but so are most of the fittings and trappings of any life, the grocery shopping and the emails and the regular visits to the dentist. I don't say this to discount the labour of care, or its demands. It's more that I had somehow thought that this could only ever be unbearable, that any and every heart would break under the strain, including those hearts that had cared for me. But none of this is true. It hurts sometimes, but that's ok.

I sometimes think about an exercise that psychologists seem to love, and that so often irritated me for how tangential it seemed to be to the point that I was making at the time. It's an exercise in kindness, although it isn't named as such, where the psychologist will meet any piece of malevolent, self-loathing trash-talk lobbied by the illness with the suggestion to respond as if it were a loved one who had said those words. And while I still think it's too simple a formulation (and very often tangential to the point), I'm also delighted by the way my girlfriend and I, we two crazy people, have somehow made their metaphor almost literal. Especially because we're both autistic (neither of us knew this when we met) and literalisation is, accordingly, something at which we both excel. But I think about it too because it also speaks to what it is we offer to each other, so unexpectedly: that recognition, which neither of us ever thought that we might ever find.

Swimming with Dolphins

Jennifer Wong

Source: A guide to what works for depression: an evidence-based review by Beyond Blue

What is it? It has been suggested that swimming with dolphins may be helpful for depression. Swimming with dolphins is usually only available through a tour operator in selected locations.

How is it meant to work? This is unclear. Dolphins use sonar signals to navigate, which could affect cell membranes in the brain. Alternatively, the natural setting or the enjoyment from the activity could also help to reduce depression.

Source: WhatsApp messages from Jennifer Wong to her mother

Hey Mum
Thanks for checking in
I'm ok
Still not feeling great
Am reading about swimming with dolphins as a way to treat depression

Dolphins?
Where are we going to get a dolphin?
Your Dad has goldfish
You want to come over and look at the goldfish?

Maybe I have to move to Queensland
To SeaWorld
Maybe my problem is I live on land too much?

I think you should try exercising
Before you try the dolphins
How about yoga?
Have you tried yoga?

Hello?

Source: To-do list

- Pick up medication
- Laundry
- Learn to swim

Source: Text messages from Jennifer Wong to swim instructor

Monday 1:12pm
Hi Liesl. It's Jennifer Wong here. I'm so sorry not to contact you earlier. Having one of those days with my depression where I can't move very much and it's taken me until now to message you. Can we please reschedule?

Monday 1:18pm
Hello Jennifer, no problem! How about tomorrow morning at 8am?

Monday 2:04pm
Thank you Liesl. See you then.

Tuesday 7:53am
Hi Liesl. I'm so, so sorry. My tendency to say yes to things without stating what my needs are, as well as the physical symptoms of my depression which make mornings very difficult has meant that I set myself up for failure yesterday when I said yes to us meeting at 8am today. I know from cognitive behavioural therapy that the use of the word 'failure' is unnecessarily harsh labelling, and that it enforces a story I tell myself about what I can and cannot do and who I am and am not. So perhaps in the spirit of a growth mindset, I can instead acknowledge that when it comes to attending early morning

appointments, there is definitely room to improve. Unfortunately my depression is so bad at the moment that I cannot tell whether it's the depression or my sensible self that's making me tell you I should postpone starting swimming lessons. I know it will be good for me in the long run, because it will mean that I can swim with dolphins, but right now I can't even leave my bed. So sorry to take up your time.

Source: Employee exit form

Name: Jennifer Wong
Reason for leaving: Office location is located inland; has limited if no proximity to ocean.

Source: A guide to what works for depression: an evidence-based review by Beyond Blue

Does it work? One study with 30 mildly-depressed adults has evaluated swimming with dolphins. Half spent one hour a day swimming and playing with bottlenose dolphins for two weeks, and the other half swam and learnt about the marine ecosystem as a control. Both groups improved, however the dolphin group improved more. Other researchers have questioned these findings. They have argued that the swimming-only group would have been disappointed to miss out on interacting with dolphins and that the disappointment made them improve less.

Source: Transcript of dolphin conversation

Flipper: Is it just me, or do you sense...a feeling of sadness amongst this bunch of people?

Snorky: I picked up on it too! I heard them described as 'mildly depressed'. Apparently today is the first day of an experiment?

Flipper: Is it an experiment to find out how we'll be affected by spending time with 30 mildly depressed adults? First we have to jump through hoops for the entertainment of humans, now we have to treat their mental health? When will humans stop leaning on the animal kingdom?

Snorky: The worst thing is that we can't even communicate how much we hate being held in captivity because our faces look like we're perpetually smiling.

Flipper: On reflection, I guess I do empathise with people who are dealing with suffering and are unable to communicate it.

Snorky: I guess…it wouldn't kill us to eat the fish they're offering…

Flipper: Who am I to swim in the way of someone wanting to improve their mental health?

Snorky: Watch out though, I get the sense that some of these guys haven't spent much time in the water before…

Source: A guide to what works for depression: an evidence-based review by Beyond Blue

Are there any risks? Swimming skills are required and there is a risk of accidental injury.

Source: Local newspaper headline

'SeaWorld dolphin injures depressed Chinese woman in freak accident'

Source: SeaWorld incident report
On the afternoon of Wednesday 16 February – conditions sunny and clear – Flipper (150-kilogram bottlenose dolphin, male) performed a routine hoop jump and landed on a participant involved in a study on swimming with dolphins as a way to alleviate depression.

The participant (70-kilogram Chinese, female), a weak swimmer, appeared absent-minded and slow to respond to instructions to clear the way for Flipper's landing. She sustained injuries to her ego from the extreme embarrassment of being knocked underwater by a large mammal, which was witnessed by 29 mildly depressed adults.

Source: Selected quotes from participant feedback forms

Male, age 53: 'I'm not sure if my depression improved, but boy it was nice to be in the sun and the water every day for two weeks. My meals were taken care of, the hotel we stayed in was nice, and I think I even got a bit of a tan…Not having to work for two weeks is also pretty sweet. Pity it's back to the grind on Monday.'

Female, age 41: 'This experience was a huge wake-up call for me to learn the skills I need for the environment I'm in. Since it's helpful to look at depression from a bio-psycho-social perspective, spending two weeks in the water with dolphins (as someone who's not confident in the water) made me think of what I need to do biologically, psychologically, and socially in order to be as at home and as comfortable as a dolphin in water.

'This has reminded me of what I learned when I went to hospital for depression…that for biological reasons I need medication and regular meals and exercise, that for psychological reasons I need therapy and to be mindful of my thinking, and for social reasons, I need to be around other people, especially when I'm depressed, even though my depression wants me to isolate. And through the cycle of recovery and relapse, it's the constant management of these things that will see me through, day to day, moment to moment.

'I'm not sure if the researchers intended for us participants to see this experience as a metaphor, but that's how I'm interpreting it. I guess you could say that one afternoon, the dolphin metaphorically and literally hit me: I am the dolphin, the water and the fish are my needs being met, and being able to play and socialise are crucial parts of being alive.'

Male, age 24: 'I have never laughed so hard as when the dolphin landed on that lady. Thank you for helping me to see the lighter side of life as well as what it looks like when someone gets absolutely pummelled by a leaping dolphin.'

Source: A guide to what works for depression: an evidence-based review by Beyond Blue

Recommendation: There is not enough good evidence to say whether swimming with dolphins works.

Source: Text messages from Jennifer Wong to swim instructor

Friday 2:37pm
Hello Liesl. I was wondering if I could try again. Do you have any afternoon beginners classes next week?

Friday 2:42pm
Great to hear from you! How about Wednesday at 2pm?

Friday 2:44pm
Thank you Liesl. See you then.

Chatterton not chatting house

Misbah Wolf

Cicada shell brooches, infectious diseases in a handful of dust,
boy-like grace conjured in blowjobs. You threatened to kill yourself
under the house. I wondered what the pattern was that connected
all living creatures. We both wrestled with Heisenberg's principle
of indeterminacy—you crouched in the dark under the house, and
me in my dressing gown on the front steps. I didn't know how fast
you were moving, and I couldn't determine your position. To survive,
I had to stop being interested in your nature. I thought about you
as a big scorpion and the remarkable fact that you would one day
have children. You told me that if I told anyone about the strategic
mapping of your suicide, you would kill yourself for certain. You
didn't think of yourself as a hunter impressed by the beauty of a
rare creature. But you were. My ribs fused with my dermal bone
expanding to protect my internal organs and my eyes just squinting
as all I could see of you was your cigarette burning down in the dark.

The Journey to Halfway

Arlea Whelan

Halfway to the frozen lake
– Frensham Little Pond –
feet lost in heather, we run
between glum firs and fronds.

Halfway to the frozen lake
– we've orders not to step out
lest we lose our breath beneath
shifting slates of ice.

Halfway to the frozen lake,
we cast ghostly gaze ashore.
No snow. No sand.
Just numb and clear and cold.

Halfway onto the frozen lake;
we've left our shoes behind
to catch the snow we know *must* fall
as these burdened days unwind.

Halfway in the frozen lake
– we're trying to catch our breath.
So many bubbles. Just one more word. Just one apology.
Just an elegy for the friends we left on the shore.

Halfway, and the frozen lake
turns our bare feet white.
Halfway, the ice closes above us.
Halfway, this is what we were warned about.
Halfway, halfway gone. Halfway, halfway home.

Halfway to the frozen lake,
we pondered, whispered and wept.

Halfway to the frozen lake,
we decided we knew best.

Halfway to the frozen lake,
we'd emptied out our chests.

Halfway to the frozen lake,
our fate was settled; our tears were fresh.

Have u a spare nut

Wart

4 my blot
for my bolt
4 my rot
for my blot

have you a spare nut for my bolt
I have a nut to screw
But I must tell you
I was never a screw
I was a slut

Didn't we all
Wots yer name
Did u 4get 22
Two
Did you
Did u too
I did
I cant remember bits
I thnk its much better
Good to 4 get

I am on your side
I am
Am I
I am
Am I

Do you distort

I have distort
Scratch sniff snuff sniff
Is it
I sit
On it
I am a sitter
Hey I can walk shit larf eat cry do upping
Is it

the absence of memory

Felicity Ward

The one thing I wish I had was a memory. I remember to turn off
the oven and to pick up my son from nursery. I remember birthdays
(thanks facebook) and lines of my stand up. But I don't remember
what depression feels like. And I don't remember what normal feels
like. And I don't remember how to hold onto joy. That is, once they're
gone.

I wasn't diagnosed with depression until I was in my thirties. But I
had some of the 'symptoms' from twenty onwards. The symptoms
that I do remember are the ones that you see on the pamphlets, on
the websites, in the movies, so I can recall them. And I remember
moments.

I remember sitting in Victoria Park. I'd just realised I was a ghost.
Like no one could hear me, and no one could see me. I couldn't feel
the sun. The traffic sound rang only in the distance. It was like I was
disappearing. I used to call it *the nothing*, like in The NeverEnding
Story. I've never actually considered until now that that's what
the film is truly about; maybe it is, maybe I'm just depressed. But
the nothing is exactly it; it consumes everything in its path and
synthesises that into nothing as well. There is a terrifying black dog
who stalks the protagonist; it growls in the darkness, it threatens
violence.

So I sat in this park, feeling nothing, not knowing what was
happening to me. I thought about going to the shops to buy some
clothes. I thought it might mean my body was doing something
normal, even if my mind wasn't. I'd had that instinct before, when
the nothingness was milder, and I did it – I bought clothes I didn't
care for, mindlessly told myself I was fine, and it had gone eventually.
But this time I chose not to; I stayed sitting on that park bench.

Feeling the swell of nothing rising up to take me. I took a pen from my bag and I slowly but firmly pressed it into my inner thigh. Maybe I could feel something then. I did. It hurt. I stopped. That wasn't the answer I was looking for. I saw a couple off to my right arguing. I thought about joining them. If they were angry, I could just walk up, punch one of them in the face, and maybe we could have a fight. That would ignite something inside me surely. That would let me feel. But I wasn't a fighter. Not a physical one anyway. So I sat there. I just sat there terrified. Waiting for my body to return.

I didn't know this was a sign of my depression until years later. I just thought it was sadness. Or being dramatic. I didn't have any language for it. I didn't know what dissociating was. I didn't know. I didn't have anyone who ever explained their depression in a way I understood. That's not true; I always thought of depression as something separate from myself so if people had said they had depression, I 'knew' in my head that I didn't have that. I thought about it as an 'other' experience.

Anxiety was much more prevalent earlier on, and much more aligned to my energy as a person. I was always described as 'hyper'. I was loud and extroverted. I loved people and conversation and dancing and singing. While this doesn't sound like the description of an anxious person, I felt like I was nearly always living life on a knife's edge. The anxiety drove the energy, the volume, the explosions of personality; it reverberated in me. And if anyone questioned it, if they told me to quiet down, or rolled their eyes, I would shatter inside. The shame was deafening. It still is, if I'm honest. I've become quieter and calmer as I've grown older – some of that is therapy and support groups and medication and exercise and meditation. But I wonder if some of it is that I just can't handle rejection? That it's still too crushing? So if I'm a little quieter, if I'm a little smaller, if I don't say what I'm angry about and just try to 'let it go' (which incidentally is me building resentments, not acceptance), then maybe they won't tell me to be quiet. Maybe they will love me. Maybe my heart won't shatter so quickly or comprehensively. Maybe it'll just be a crack.

The anxiety became too much. The constant stress. The peaking of adrenal glands. The heart racing. The sweats. The clenched jaw. The long slow rise of anxiety, coming at me like a tsunami wave. Or the instant emergency handle, ordering a code red to every nerve in my body. And then developing a soldier-like readiness for it to strike at any time. It drove me to get support. And as I've listed above, I've just about done it all.

I've had a very difficult two years, coinciding with the birth of my son, who now holds no rival to the person I love dearest and most in this world. I fall in love with him every day. I can't believe this Disney bear/elf/baby lives with me and thinks I'm his best bet. But it wasn't always like that. I had postnatal depression for the best part of a year, followed by some good old-fashioned depression on and off for the year after that. And because the two years have been so additionally difficult for so many reasons (death, family illness, the pandemic, getting covid, family injury, over-responsibility, going back to work too soon after a baby, chronic homesickness, the most overcast December in London for fifty years) I don't know how much is depression (some of it, definitely) and how much is a really bad run. Is this who I am, or would anyone feel like this?

I'm forty-one now. I can describe all these experiences, these symptoms, these memories. But I don't recognise them when they're happening to me. It's so subtle. So incremental. How can we know ourselves differently from one day to the next? It's like asking ourselves to identify how our baby has changed overnight. Do they have another hair? Can they reach higher than yesterday? It's impossible. It's a gut instinct more than anything. I am still shocked that I don't know that I'm sinking sometimes. I don't know depression is coming or happening. I think I'm fine. Just a bit tired. I wonder why people are starting to piss me off more. Why people aren't doing their jobs better. Why no one seems courteous. My body starts to ache more. I frown more often. My temper is shorter. I love less. I smile for shorter bursts. I'm wound tighter. It changes so subtly, I just realise I feel like I have ball-bearings sewn into the lining of my skin. I'm heavy. My eyes are heavy. My chest is heavy. When I'm in it, I don't know that *that* isn't my natural state. I don't know that I've lived happier, more easily, more loosely, more energised, optimistically before. I...don't remember.

I had this idea for a film where a woman lived her life but when she went to sleep she had a completely different life. She never slept, but that wasn't a problem. She just had two entirely different lives she was living. And by halfway through the film, she wasn't sure which was the dream and which was reality. That's how I feel about my mental illness: when I'm depressed I, in my maudlin state, accept with resignation that this is actually who I am – tired, sad, numb, separate from everyone and from my body, unmotivated, unfixable, existing – and that the times I feel 'happy' are the aberration. The blips. The sunny breaks in an otherwise cloudy life. At the same time, when I'm happy and light and joyous and brilliant and child-like and powerful and spirited and warm and loving, I think 'no *this* is the true me. That depression is the thing that needs to be kept at bay.'

What I haven't accepted is that both parts are the real me. The brilliance and the numbness. The loudness and the deafening silence. And if they could hold hands long enough to understand each other, then maybe I wouldn't still be fighting this damp, suffocating disease. Maybe I wouldn't hold such contempt for it, and wouldn't shove it in my own face as a victimless badge of honour.

So I wish I had a memory. I wish I remembered *me*. I wish I had a way I could look and feel how I used to be, to know that it can be different – I want to be able to smell a swimming costume I wore in my Nan's pool as I did a backflip in front of my older cousins, and have it trigger the feeling of contentment. I want a body memory of depression so I know. I want a yardstick, a photo of my heart's happiness. A cloud of depression I could keep in a jar, in my bathroom cabinet, like a medicine I might need in the future. Just something to remember me by.

Rewind. Erase. Record.

Or, fragments from a steroid-induced psychosis – 2007.

Susie Walsh

i.
There was a moment when I knew I was moving into another realm.

> *Does everyone who is going mad have this moment? Of terror?*
> *Unable to halt the inexorable? Just hoping they will come back?*
> *Will I come back from there?*

ii.
In the days beforehand there were signs.
Micro-managing
the making of my takeaway tea
from the cafe up the road.
Burying a coin
in the municipal garden beds
so I would always have enough money.
Shambolic and dishevelled,
I show the woman at a clothing shop my university ID card.

> *See, I have a job. I am capable. I am not mad.*

iii.
I. Am. Invincible. Gigantic. Magnificent.
I clean the outside front of the house. At 3am. By hand.
I do not sleep. I do not sleep. I. Do. Not. Need. Sleep.
Fearless. In the park, playing on the equipment, well after midnight.
The weed-smoking couple ask if I need
somewhere to stay for the night.
I have a home. I am not mad.
They are kind, and high.
But sceptical.

iv.

I become. Infuriated. By the colour red.
I must gather up all the red coloured things in the house and
hide them out of sight.
I become. Fixated. On the colour green.
I wander around the house clutching a handful of frozen peas.

v.

Visitations. Hallucinations.
An arm of the girl in 'Arabesque', the John Brack print, moves.
Her arm is moving. She is pointing me that way. Go that way.
Go there. Go there. Go there.

vi.

The doctor is called. The ambulance is called.
I refuse to get into the ambulance.
The police are called. *Why are the police here?*
They can fuck right off. I am not mad. Eventually.
Coaxed. Into the ambulance. I flirt with the female ambulance officer.

vii.

Please rewind this. Please erase this. Please do not record this.
I do not want to be remembered this way when I come back.
From where? Will I come back?

viii.

I point at the jumper being worn by a woman who looks in charge.
I scream:
Who the fuck wears a red jumper in an emergency department?
I point at the green exit sign.
I plead:
Home. Go there. Go home. Rewind. Rewind. Rewind.

ix.

Uncooperative. Capacity diminished. Sectioned. *I. Am. Not. Mad.*

x.

Lumbar punctured. Psychosis punctured.

xi.

Sleep. At last. Erase. Erase. *The self. The shame. The stigma.*
Erase. Erase. Erase.

xii.

Morning. Reality. Unable to go home. Not until.
The neurologist who mismanaged me reviews and releases me. *What?*
I go outside to the hospital grounds to think before he arrives. *Fuck.*
How am I going to prove that I am sane? Why do I have to do that?
Fuck him.

xiii.

It takes immense effort to not use pressured speech.
To not be angry with him.

> *Be calm. Be rational. Be amenable. Be compliant.*
> *Be sane for fuck's sake. Be sane.*

xiv.

Discharged. With paperwork proving my sanity.
Might come in handy one day.

> Rewind. Erase. Record. Record. Record *this* moment.
> *Just this moment.*

xv.

Over the following days and weeks. Or is it months?
There are slippages, and reminders:

> A red wastepaper basket filled with other red things
> hidden in the linen cupboard.
> Desiccated peas in odd places.

What if I had not come back from there? Rewind. Erase. Record.
Record it all.

Memories sometimes come backwards

Ellen van Neerven

Memories sometimes come backwards. They haunt-walk in.
My therapist – in our last session together before she left – asked
me to describe the creative process. I said a voice to throw belief
at. How I sit at one side of the table to tip tap on the laptop and the
other to write in my notebook. This morning I faced an identity crisis
organising my wardrobe. It is mid-spring and I'm not yet warm. In
my home, my Country – now several hundred kilometres north-east
from here – the sun sits on my shoulders. Every breath is a loss
or gain of water. Here, my legs curl to my knees and my throat is
always dry.

Memories sometimes come backwards. They haunt-walk in.
Haunting, walking, and sugar from the chocolates my friends give me
after 'the incident'. 'We are in great admiration of how you handled
yourself. We thought you conducted yourself with such dignity
and grace.' I did nothing but lie in my bed. As I search for a card in
the chocolate box, something tells me I'm not meant to hear about
what people think about me – this kind of aggrieved love – until I'm
dead. So I'm walking-dead-haunting-live and there seems nothing
left to do but write about my trauma. My therapist has left and I
haven't done my hw for my osteo. My inbox is full of sympathy and
unsympathetic requests.

Memories sometimes come backwards. They haunt-walk in.
Writing around trauma is easy when the commissions keep coming.
I'm flirting with myself, my reflection in the glass door does not
need to ask for my number. My laptop screen greens with displeased
fingers. After 'the incident' my gf spends time weeding my emails, we
are e-entwined. If I get a +ve one I promise to respond in 2–30 days.
If I get a –ve one I promise to screenshot.

Preface to *The Rapids*

Sam Twyford-Moore

In 2018, as I was putting the finishing touches to my book *The Rapids: Ways of Looking at Mania* – a sometimes uneasy mix of close memoir and broad cultural criticism – one of its subjects disrupted the narrative sequence I was completing in my head. Kanye West dropped his anticipated album *Ye* on the first day of winter as I powered through final proof pages. It wasn't the music per se that stopped my workflow. Rather, it was its striking cover – deliberately designed as a talk-piece – that halted my momentum. According to a tweet from his then-wife, Kim Kardashian West, Kanye took the photograph of the album's cover – a purple Wyoming mountain-scape at dusk – while in transit to the record's debut at a listening party. The final artwork featured lime green text scrawled across that photo, Kanye broadcasting the showstopper message: 'I hate being Bi-Polar its awesome'.

Just as its cover perfectly captured the contradictory nature of the condition widely known as bipolarity, the record featured lyrics with direct references to the disorder, including a powerful cut-through statement that he saw the condition as a 'superpower' rather than a disability.

My publisher understandably emailed to see if I wanted to update the text of the book to reflect this new perspective from Yeezy, but I was so very late in the edits and so weary from revisiting my own 'superpower/disability' confessions that I couldn't pull together the energy to do so. How very un-Kanye of me, you might say (doubly so, given Kanye's infamous last-minute tinkering with projects and his perfectionism).

This unexpected disruption, however, points to the ever-evolving nature of conversations around mental ill-health. A writer needs to realise that they can't always keep up and that the static-ness of any finished work can never really capture shifting ground. It can offer instead a record – a marker – of where the conversation about its subject is at the time of its writing. But even that record is never entirely fixed in place. A writer is invited, after all, to talk about a finished work on panels at festivals and in the media, and it seems to me that it is here, at these appearances, that the real thinking begins.

Here is one instance. Sitting on a panel with a writer who had recently been diagnosed with bipolar, with tears in their eyes, they sat looking out at the audience and posed a frank question: 'What becomes of joy? What is elation to you when you have issues with controlling an elevated mood?' I had been experiencing a similar feeling of confusion, though in my case this related to being able to tell the difference between lashing out during a manic episode and standing up for myself when not in that emotionally unstable state. I had negotiated this complicated field after *The Rapids* was released. The book proved to be something of a lightning rod when published. One imagines most nonfiction books are ideally just that – conversation starters, provocations, polemics – and that they can act as little hand grenades lobbed from a safe enough distance. They aren't thrown in glee. I didn't know quite what I was in for. Certainly, I did not feel that this was a particularly provocative book – it definitely wasn't a Kanye-stumping-for-Trump act of contrarianism – and yet, a once-close friend emailed me to say I 'did not deserve' – and, more to the point, 'had no right' – to publish the book, making strained claims that I had not done enough work to vet the book with people in proximity to my manic episodes. The email came out of nowhere and knocked me flat. With its strong language and the fact it hit my inbox the week the book hit the shelves, it only added to my pre-existing pre-release anxiety. I shouldn't have been so surprised, perhaps. People turn. The email had a particular sting to it, however, because it felt like such a keen example of stigma in action. I was hoping to eradicate that kind of response with the internal dialogue within the book, but I had not accounted for people responding without having read it at all.

When I received the contract to write my book, I made a conscious decision not to spend more than a year working on it. I explained to friends at the time that the topic was too heavy to live with for any longer than that. There already feels like there is a radioactive-like half-life to manic episodes – no need to extend them any further by writing for years on the topic, I thought. There are, after all, the ongoing material conditions that you must live in the years after. There are the losses of once-close friendships. There are the damages to your reputation. There are the financial implications of past transgressions.

It is, however, possible as you move away in time from your last episode – manic or depressive –to simply forget that the condition resides inside you. Indeed, treatment can provide an incredible sense of stability, but it can also make the illness invisible to oneself. The need to narrativise, or to consider the cultural implications of your diagnosis, can recede too. Writing essays such as these has always served as a reminder not to become complacent about living with the disorder, as it refocuses me on a central question that has been there all along: what is mania as a cultural identity and what is a psychiatric disability that can disappear from daily life with treatment? If you're not projecting outward, how can you ever be seen?

*

In Whit Stillman's masterpiece *The Last Days of Disco*, Chloë Sevigny's romantic interest Josh talks openly about his experiences with manic depression. In Stillman's typically sharp, purposefully stilted dialogue, Josh observes that he finds a friend's nickname for him – 'loon' – endearing, whereas other terms – 'nutcase' and 'freakazoid' – get to him. Josh likes 'loon' because it's both short for lunatic and the 'lakebird with the eerie call', which might sound twee, but his sensitivity to nomenclature is shared with many diagnosed with this unstable disorder. The same observation about preferences for designated terminology was played more as an outright gag in Tim Robinson's underseen sitcom *Detroiters*. Robinson's father is a mythic ad man of yore in the series and the only other thing we know about him is that he has been institutionalised after having a breakdown in the middle of a business meeting. An old colleague tells Robinson that he knew his father and was actually in the meeting where he 'you know...went nuts'. Robinson stops the colleague and stonily explains that, when it comes to his father, he prefers to use the term 'bonkers'. My wife and I quote that particular phrasing regularly to each other. (Moments of humour are an integral part of ongoing survival.)

I document these cultural recollections as a way of saying that the language relating to the disorder is ever changing. When writing *The Rapids*, I couldn't keep clear in my mind whether to call it a disorder, disease, illness or condition. Perhaps it was all of these and perhaps none. I would type one and then delete the other. I was distressed when my friend, in sending that harsh post-publication email, repeatedly referred to my 'illness'. It was a 'condition' I protested, but then I had referred to it as an 'illness' many times over myself.

This was all unfolding while, in the background, the phrase 'lived experience' was breaking through and with it a significant cultural discussion about prioritising books and essays about subjects from people who have lived through them from a subjective perspective. This was extremely useful in terms of having a way to frame my book when talking about it in public. Ultimately, I believe that how a book is framed is decided by its readers. More than one commented to me that the book was 'quite chatty'. (I can possibly be 'quite chatty' on social media too, and if I ever have another manic episode, I hope someone takes my accounts and passwords away from me, as they amplify the worst of the public expressions of the disorder.) This felt appropriate given a chapter is given over to exploring the effects of compulsive speech in mania. Indeed, the book seemed to take on many of the traits of what it discussed. One of the unintended consequences of the style of broken nonfiction *The Rapids* is written in, for instance, is that some readers with past experiences of dissociative disorders noted having had transference-like experiences from reading the text. This was certainly not my intention (I joked that I had considered asking my publisher to include a warning sticker, 'May induce mild mania' as a way to promote sales.)

In all my writing on mental ill-health to date, there might have been an underlying intention – conscious or otherwise – to create work which reads as chaotically and incoherently as the condition in question. Writing about depression might be flat and expressionless; writing about mania may be just as choppy and changey as its disrupted moods. These acts of mirroring contain an obvious desire to express how it feels to live with mental ill health. In which case, questions of the qualitative type should be rendered useless. Your criticism doesn't really matter. It is my sincere hope that the reader knows they bear some responsibility, that they are to do some of the work, and that their thinking must bring the clarity the writing is asking for, wanting, and ultimately deserves.

Diorama, retrospective

Lindsay Tuggle

Some acts are chosen.
Others choose you.

Aftermaths are as personal as fingerprints.
Drunken ghosts downpour maledictions

until we hunt machines of our own creation,
make cathedrals of our bitten selves.

Just imagine the bruises the fall must have caused.

That afternoon I saw another doctor
to milk a wound for all its worth.

No pretty utterances on the couch
only gutter glass and all my best vintage,

The clothes that guard against your eyes.

Alterity is underwhelming.
Sometimes 'no' is the only word a mouth can shape.

My criminal record includes truancy
which is simply a refusal to remain in the designated place.

Always, this compulsion to run until the femur cracks.
When I was thirteen we lived in the woods for four nights.

We slept on beds of leaves,
ribs curled into fists around our hearts.

We fled because we didn't want to wed the holy ghost.
Or any ghost, for that matter.

We were destined for evergreens, slow leavings,
the fleeting joy of feeling almost safe.

Night fell softly on limbs untouched by animal husbandry,
before the bridal elegy began.

Smart Ovens for Lonely People

Elizabeth Tan

After that day at the overpass I was assigned an oven. It was manufactured by a company known for its cutting-edge cuteness. This oven was called Neko Oven because it was shaped like a giant cat's head. It had a rounded chamber, a triangular-eared hood, and an alarm that sounded very much like the jingle of a cat's bell.

The oven was covered by my insurance. Let me be clear, though: my Neko Oven was not at all like those gauche models featured in the commercials, the ones in which sexily deep-voiced ovens whisper/bake sweet nothings for sad single people. Neko Oven was quite classy actually. She (for Neko Oven was programmed with a female voice) was fond of kindly but firmly stating the limits of her responsibilities. *THAT IS NOT MY FUNCTION*, she'd say when I would ask her if she thought I was ready to unblock Adam from my newsfeed, or whether she could recommend any forms of self-harm that were relatively harmless, like holding ice cubes. *THAT IS NOT MY FUNCTION*, she would say sedately, and then, *WOULD YOU LIKE SOME SHEPHERD'S PIE?*

No, nobody could accuse Neko Oven of being an enabler. Because she couldn't do everything by herself. For the first week she just sat in my kitchen in her cat-shaped cardboard carton. There's no way to guarantee that a person assigned their oven will actually even get around to activating it. Perhaps there's some smug clinical reasoning for that, like: in order for recovery to work, the client must independently arrive at a place where they are ready to accept help. To peel back that first strip of packing tape from the box.

That was the day of Lydia's disastrous kitchen tea. It turns out that your love for a dear friend does not negate the crushing tedium of having to study the minutiae of her courtship with her future husband. Because Lydia had decided that in order to control the queue for the buffet she would require guests to first complete some kind of diabolical Sudoku–crossword hybrid puzzle about her and her fiancé. 1, Across: Where did Lydia and Liam meet? 2, Down: What did Lydia and Liam eat on their first date? 3, Across: What is the date of Lydia and Liam's dating anniversary? 4, Down: What is the date of Lydia and Liam's engagement anniversary?

On and on and on. That was the day I learnt, via Lydia's aunt, how to say 'This is bullshit' in French (*C'est des conneries*). Perhaps it was this lingering kinship with the puckered aunt's *crise de colère* that compelled me to finally set up Neko Oven.

And that was it – the hard part, over. Neko Oven awoke with three crisp bell notes, synced herself with the fridge and pantry, and asked me to grate two carrots, please. The first meal she made for me was a frittata. A frittata is typically one of the first meals a smart oven makes for you because it's easy to hide vegetables and stale ingredients in the egg mixture. It was a golden, hopeful start to our relationship: Neko Oven was going to take my meagre, wilted scraps and turn them into something silky and nutritious.

Just like her feline namesake, Neko Oven was self-cleaning. I sat at the kitchen table reading her instruction manual and the terms of her hire period as she rumbled softly through her wash cycle. I was covered for one year with Neko Oven, with the potential for an extension of another six months pending a progress report from Neko Oven herself.

WOULD YOU LIKE ME TO PLAY SOME LIGHT MUSIC? Neko Oven asked once she was done sloshing herself with sudsy water. She played a little sample of 'God Only Knows' by The Beach Boys, but, due to licensing issues, she rendered it entirely with her little range of bell sounds.

'I'm sorry I took so long to unpack you,' I said.

IT'S OKAY, she said. And then:

YOU DON'T HAVE TO BE SORRY ANYMORE.

*

I ended up discarding most of the frittata leftovers. Neko Oven didn't say a word about it, and would never say a word about anything I wasted, and I learned, just like she said on that first night, not to be sorry all the time.

Adam heard about what happened and arranged to meet me for coffee. He came straight from rehearsal and he was still wearing his character's clothes, a dress shirt and pressed suit pants and suspenders. I had arrived unwisely early and was already seated when he showed – perhaps it was up to me to rise and hug him in greeting, but I didn't. He stacked his phone and keys on the table and I caught sight, then, of an unfamiliar ornament on his keychain: a mini silver Eiffel Tower. My mind itched with speculations.

'How are you?' he asked in that hushed cautious voice everyone was using around me.

'Okay,' I said. 'How are you?'

And, relieved, he told me about his new production, repeating facts that he'd forgotten he'd already told me, and he kept saying, 'I feel like I'm really pushing myself as an actor.' He sat close to the edge of his seat as if he was only going to stay for a minute, and he kept reviving his phone to check the time, and I kept pretending not to notice. He smelled of muscular body spray and car upholstery.

And once the warm-up talk was over it was time for him to say: 'So. You almost died.'

'Yeah.'

I felt once again the rush of morning traffic, the arms of a stranger.

And what was that look, in Adam's eyes? Actual sadness? Or a kind of perfunctory empathy, the detection of a blip in his beautiful universe, something to rectify as soon as possible so he could keep sailing on?

He asked if I was still getting therapy. If I was still living alone. If Lydia was looking after me, if my mother was looking after me, if Biljana and the others at work knew about what happened. Perhaps he wanted to reassure himself that he didn't have to do more than this one coffee meeting, a quick hour between appointments.

'I'm glad you're doing better now, Shu,' he said.

He checked his phone again and this time I noticed that the background of his lock screen was a selfie of him with his arm around a woman I'd never seen before. Coldness crept over me.

There wasn't much more to say after that. Adam said he had to go, and when he crossed the street to his car his eyes were already on his phone, swiping a text message. He drove off without looking back.

*

On the way home I bought frozen peas, mini Roma tomatoes, beef mince close to expiry. I bought Dutch cream potatoes, dried pasta shells, chicken stock cubes, jasmine rice.

PLEASE PEEL SEVEN POTATOES, Neko Oven said.

PLEASE DICE THE POTATOES INTO CUBES.

PLEASE PLACE THE POTATOES IN A SAUCEPAN OF SALTY WATER.

PLEASE PLACE THE SAUCEPAN ON MY LEFT BURNER.

I was doing what psychologists call *ruminating*. I was *indulging in unhelpful thinking*. I was listening to a mixtape I'd made for Adam back when we were dating. The theme of the mixtape was hugging and included songs like 'Throw Your Arms Around Me' by Hunters & Collectors. I wasted all of the best hugging songs on a relationship that lasted less than a year.

DO YOU KNOW THE DIFFERENCE BETWEEN A SHEPHERD'S PIE AND A COTTAGE PIE?

'No.'

A SHEPHERD'S PIE IS TRADITIONALLY MADE WITH MINCED LAMB OR MUTTON, WHEREAS A COTTAGE PIE IS TRADITIONALLY MADE WITH MINCED BEEF. SO ACTUALLY WE ARE MAKING A COTTAGE PIE.

They looked to be near the Swan River, at a wedding, perhaps – Adam was wearing a tie and there were white chairs in the background of the lock screen photo. Their eyes were small from the sunlight; they were smiling. How did they meet? How long had they been together? Who was getting married – a cousin of Adam's, perhaps? He never invited me to family events when we were dating. He never changed his lock screen to a photo of us.

PLEASE DICE ONE ONION FINELY.

PLEASE CUT THE MINI ROMA TOMATOES INTO QUARTERS.

There was a pile of laundry that needed washing; there were stiff clothes hanging on the collapsible washing line I'd set up in the living room a week ago. I hadn't changed my bedsheets for nearly three months, which meant they were the same sheets I'd slept in on that day at the overpass. Everywhere there seemed to be indictments of my failure to meet some low bar of adulthood – fallen hair coiled in drain holes, unopened bills, white dried spots of toothpaste on the bathroom counter.

PLEASE SEASON THE MINCE WITH SALT AND PEPPER.

PLEASE FRY THE ONION IN A LITTLE BIT OF OLIVE OIL.

Was she working on the same production as him? Was she an actress, a lighting technician, a stage manager? How soon after breaking up with me did he meet her? Is she funnier than me? Is she better at sex than me? Did she know he met me for coffee that day? Did she pity me?

'Those same damn bottles going out and those same damn bottles coming back.'

PARDON?

I froze. I wondered what would happen if I didn't respond to Neko Oven – whether she would just ask the same question again and again.

'Sorry. That's just something I say sometimes. When I'm having repetitive thoughts. Because I feel like I'm a survivor on a deserted island, throwing messages in glass bottles into the sea, only for the tide to keep bringing them back. *Those same damn bottles going out and those same damn bottles coming back.*'

I wondered if Neko Oven had any notion of survivors on deserted islands. If a machine understood loneliness, or repetitive thoughts, or talking to oneself.

I SEE.

And then, hopefully:

SO YOU SAY THIS PHRASE IN THE MANNER OF A MANTRA?

I smiled. 'Kind of like a mantra, yeah.'

*

After Neko Oven had been activated for two weeks she sent a recommendation to Biljana to let me return to work. Biljana gave me a hug when I arrived at the shop, a rare gesture, and it was strange to discover that underneath those billowy kaftans was a small sculpted body. She let me focus on alterations all day and jumped up to attend to customers before I could even lift my eyes from my machine.

On my lunchbreak I used the kitchenette microwave to heat up a little plastic container of Neko Oven's leftovers (some kind of casserole she'd improvised from tinned chickpeas, bacon, and gin) and took it to the food court to eat alone. It was nearly two o'clock, so the food court was empty except for cappuccino-sipping seniors and other workers on their lunchbreaks, their uniform hats or aprons scrunched up in their laps, scrolling through their newsfeeds, squeezing black drops of soy sauce onto their sushi from little fish-shaped tubes.

I was doing that mindfulness thing that my psychologist told me to do – where I would notice five things I could see, five things I could hear, five things I could feel – when I heard someone say: 'Shu?'

And there was Lydia, holding a lacquered wooden ampersand and two lacquered wooden *L*s that she'd just purchased from Typo.

I stood up, and she put her wooden letters down on the table and flung her arms around me. She said she was sorry we didn't get the chance to talk properly at the kitchen tea, and that she'd still love for me to be a bridesmaid, but after what happened she didn't want to make demands on me, but also she didn't want me to think that she thought that I couldn't handle the commitment of being a bridesmaid.

Also, Liam had already asked three of his friends to be groomsmen and she really wanted the sides to be even so if I couldn't be a bridesmaid she'll have to ask somebody else because it'd be awkward to demote a groomsman after they've all already said yes and put down deposits on matching suits.

'No, of course, I understand,' I said. 'And I'm happy to be your bridesmaid. For sure.' I was about to apologise for stressing her out, but then I remembered that Neko Oven said I didn't need to be sorry anymore.

'Good. Oh, good. I'm so glad.' And then Lydia's eyes softened. I braced myself. 'And how *are* you?' she asked. 'Back at work today?'

I told her that I was in the smart oven program. I pointed at my lunch with pride. Lydia clapped appreciatively. She asked me what model I had, so I told her about Neko Oven. I described her cat-shaped hood and her bell sounds and her sedate non-judgemental voice.

'Oh, Shu!' Lydia exclaimed. 'That's just wonderful.'

And then she said: 'You know, it's like I've always said: living all by yourself, all alone in that apartment – you really need a cat. A really cute cat. So you won't be lonely. So you'll have some company.' Lydia smiled. 'And now you have one.'

*

'It's just patronising, that's all,' I said to Neko Oven later while I was separating the squashed mini Roma tomatoes from the firmer ones. 'She always used to suggest I get a pet cat. Whenever she'd ask how I was going and I'd say that I was lonely or I missed Adam or I hadn't talked to anybody besides customers for three days straight.'

Neko Oven blinked her lights speculatively, but didn't say anything. She adjusted the heat on one of her burners.

'I mean – she doesn't *mean* it to be patronising. She doesn't know that she's saying something that I get all the time. Especially from people who are in relationships already. That's the thing. It only ever comes from people who are happily coupled off. *Why don't you get a cat, Shu?* Then they go off on their date nights and upload gorgeous photos to Instagram.'

PLEASE SLICE THE MINI ROMA TOMATOES INTO HALVES, Neko Oven said, so I did.

'Should I tell Lydia not to say things like that? What do you think I should do?'

THAT IS NOT MY FUNCTION.

Of course.

I concentrated on the sound of the knife hitting the bottom of the chopping board. The acidic fragrance of overripe tomatoes.

BUT IT IS TRUE WHAT YOU SAY, Neko Oven conceded. THERE ARE LIMITATIONS TO THE CARE THAT A PET OR A SMART OVEN CAN PROVIDE TO A HUMAN.

She started to ping out a song with her bell tones. At first I thought she was ad-libbing, but then I figured out that the tune was 'Wuthering Heights' by Kate Bush, which had absolutely no relevance to the discussion at hand. She was always doing things like that. I kept thinking about Lydia. I wanted absurdly to make her feel bad for making me feel bad.

THOSE SAME DAMN BOTTLES GOING OUT, Neko Oven said.

Those same damn bottles coming back.

I'd had Neko Oven for about three months when I saw the stranger again. We were waiting on opposite platforms at the train station, the only two people there. There was no uncertainty, no double-takes – we knew immediately. He was even wearing the same grey-and-green striped hoodie which had caught my eye that fateful morning. For a moment we just looked at each other from across the tracks; he lifted his hand in a sheepish wave. Then he picked up his shopping bags, climbed the stairs, and crossed over to my platform. 'It's good to see you again,' he said.

'It's good to see you too,' I said, which was the truth, even though I was embarrassed.

'I never said thank you,' he said, 'for what you did that day.'

'I never said thank you either,' I said.

He smiled a little. 'What are the odds? Two people choosing the same overpass to jump from. The same time, the same day.'

'Yeah.'

We stood next to each other for a long time. An abandoned babycino cup was rocking back and forth on the train tracks, a thin smile of chocolate stuck to the bottom.

'Would you say that you're okay now?' I asked the stranger.

'Would you?'

'No.'

'No.'

'*The next train to – Perth – departs in – five minutes,*' came the announcement, but, with the stranger next to me, I couldn't help but hear the announcement in Neko Oven's melodious and measured voice. I wondered if we should even be talking to each other.

'Still,' the stranger said, 'I guess we keep going.'

His voice creaked like the broken spine of a Bible. One of his fraying green shopping bags contained baked beans, bananas, dried spaghetti, tinned tuna, and as he rearranged his grip on the handles I noticed he was wearing a wedding ring. The sight of it zapped me, a truth I'd always known: having someone who loves you doesn't exempt you from wanting to die.

'The worst thing,' he said, as if he heard my last thought, 'is not being able to explain why.'

Why.

Why.

When people asked, 'How *are* you?' did they really mean, '*Why* did you?'

His train was about to arrive, so we said goodbye. He climbed the stairs, lifting his legs in a broken gait that I recognised in myself, the green shopping bags sagging, as if they, too, were ready for things to end.

*

Because I was tired.

Because I wanted to die, the same way you might want a drink of water, or want to sleep, or want someone to love you back.

Because staying alive took so much work. All that searching oneself for the problem, fumbling for a way to articulate the problem; all that getting out of bed, sliding into cold clothes, spooning cereal from bowl to mouth.

And the appointments. A doctor and a trail of invoices for every failing part of me – eyes, skin, brain, teeth, waistline, uterus, heart.

Because I realised that it was my biological imperative to die, that dying was my body's default function. My whole body, conspiring to die, dedicated to the task of dying.

Because I was bored. Because it was boring to sleep. Because it was boring to retell the story to each new therapist, crisis hotline operator, psychiatrist. Because listening to the same guided meditation tracks was boring. Because the compulsive dragged thumb, hold, release, refresh on an inert newsfeed was boring. Because crying was boring. Because being unable to cry was boring. Because the white walls and bedsheets and the hollowed indent in the mattress were boring.

Because I couldn't call anybody, even though that's what people say – *you can call me anytime*. To say what? I am bored? I am sad? I want to die?

Because I'd tried therapy. I'd tried escitalopram, duloxetine, desvenlafaxine. I'd tried phoning a friend. I'd tried Pilates and focusing on the breath. I'd tried being curious about my feelings. I'd tried thinking of five things I was grateful for. I'd tried thinking: the sky is blue, the grass is green.

But I hadn't tried dying.

*

I told Neko Oven about meeting the stranger from the overpass as I was slicing an eggplant. We were making Moussaka. She didn't interrupt me at all, just blinked her lights occasionally to let me know that she was listening.

How do you feel about the encounter? she asked when I was finished.

'I don't know. I don't know if it did any good.'

Conversations do not need to do good or bad. They can just be conversations.

'That's true.'

If we were to apply your metaphor about messages inside bottles, we could say that you discovered new bottles on the shore of your solitary island, a fresh reminder that there are other islands and other people throwing bottles, that while you are alone on your island you are not alone in the ocean.

'I guess so.'

Such a reminder is neither good nor bad. It is just information.

A neutral fact.

The ocean is full of bottles.

That is why I and others like me exist.

It is time to fry the eggplant.

I placed the frying pan on her left burner. I drizzled olive oil into the pan. 'How long on average do people need their smart oven?' I asked.

IT IS DIFFICULT TO ANSWER YOUR QUESTION ACCURATELY, said Neko Oven.

SOME CLIENTS MUST RETURN THEIR SMART OVEN BEFORE THEY HAVE MADE A FULL RECOVERY.

SOME CLIENTS ONLY USE THEIR SMART OVEN FOR TWO TO FOUR WEEKS.

SOME CLIENTS ARE STABLE FOR MANY MONTHS BUT THEN UNDERGO A RELAPSE IN THE FINAL WEEK OF THEIR HIRE PERIOD.

SOME CLIENTS LEAVE THE SMART OVEN PROGRAM AND THEN RETURN INTERMITTENTLY.

She paused. Was Neko Oven really thinking, whenever she paused like that? Wouldn't a machine as smart as her take less than one second to formulate a response to me? Was the pause for my benefit?

She continued:

YOU COULD SAY THAT THE PROBLEM IS:

(1) THE IMPOSSIBILITY OF QUANTIFYING NEED; AND

(2) THE NON-LINEARITY OF RECOVERY.

*

The day that Lydia and Liam got married was as picturesque and luscious as it was foretold by Lydia's Pinterest board. The ribbons on the bridesmaids' bouquets matched the colours of the groomsmen's bowties, and as I stood watching my friend glide down the aisle towards a life we'd been taught to want and probably did genuinely want I found that I could be both desperately lonely and profoundly happy; I could always be both.

After the ceremony, I clasped a basket of mini-quiches that Neko Oven helped me to prepare so that the bridal party would have something to eat during the photo shoot. The groomsmen and the other bridesmaids were particularly enthused about the way the crust didn't crumble and scatter pastry everywhere, and I couldn't wait to pass on the compliment to Neko Oven.

Lydia really got her money's worth out of those giant wooden letters: the L & L appeared in almost every photo – gathered in Lydia and Liam's arms as they kissed, tangled in Lydia's veil in an overhead shot of Lydia and Liam lying on the lawn, propped on the ground as the bride and her bridesmaids leapt and tossed their bouquets in the air.

Between shooting locations, when nearly all the mini-quiches were gone, Lydia caught my hand and asked how I was going. 'Maybe this is silly of me but I'll be relieved when this is all over,' Lydia said. 'All this – this shouldn't be life.'

'I suppose not,' I said.

This close, she appeared so much like my old friend, only rendered with more vibrant brushstrokes. 'Listen, Shu,' Lydia said, clasping my hand again. The wedding ring gave her hand a new weight. 'I love you so much. I'm so glad you're here.'

I could tell she meant that last part in every single way that the sentence could be meant. She summoned the photographer to take a picture of just us together, and then she went off to join Liam.

I took one of the last mini-quiches from the basket. It fit so neatly in my hand, this golden vessel; I spied a sundried tomato buried like a jewel close to the surface of the pillow-soft filling. What is the difference between a quiche and a frittata? I made a mental note to ask Neko Oven as I took a bite. It really was true, what everyone was saying: Neko Oven did a fantastic job with the crust.

How To Be Happy
Cher Tan

There is no such thing as unbridled joy. Sometimes it appears, fleeting. She intellectually recognises it. She understands what it means in the abstract. But what is joy? She does not know.

For a long time she did not know what it meant to be sick in the brain; she thought it was merely a part of her personality; a quirk, an idiosyncrasy. It could still very well be. Age five, senselessly destroying schoolmates' artwork out of boredom, only to be chastised and locked in a broom closet for hours. She couldn't stop screaming. Age nine, repeatedly pressing a doorbell at a stranger's house near her school to see how it worked, only to receive punishment later for being a troublemaker. Age fourteen, targeted by classmates who saw her as a snob because she was ostensibly 'clever', but did not know how to socialise. Age seventeen, getting kicked out of school for stealing, again, out of boredom, and perhaps some subconscious need – for money, for care, for attention. Age twenty, almost extinguishing her life. She nearly did not finish high school. She cannot seem to hold down a job. And on and on and on. Today at age thirty-five she still cannot read others' expressions or emotions, even her boyfriend whom she has been with for nearly a decade. I'm sure people still regard her as a snob. She cries perhaps once every two years. She is unable to express anger, or excitement, or disappointment, a lot of which appear externally as a flat affect. Usually she takes to masking: she knows how these feelings are meant to appear – sort of. Two become one; one manifests and it is convincing. Congratulations! I'm so happy for you.

What came first: the conditions for mental illness to develop, or a broken brain that then results in conditions which cause mental illness to develop? She knows all the medical words. For years she pored through books – often in private – to try and solve the mystery of her brain. She's read several memoirs (she barely reads memoirs): they all seem to come with these rough-to-the-touch matte covers, often with a picture of the author on the front, some piss-weak design, and exist within the strange dichotomy of high GSM pages or extremely flimsy ones. And they never usually smell that good. It's one of those things that's incorrigibly gauche unless you relate to its contents; maybe that's how they're pulling it off nowadays with novels. In *The Unquiet Mind*, Kay Redfield Jamison writes, 'I did not wake up one day to find myself mad. Life should be so simple.' Temple Grandin, in *Thinking in Pictures*, points out that she gets 'great satisfaction out of doing clever things with my mind, but I don't know what it is like to feel rapturous joy.' And Sascha Altman DuBrul, in *Navigating the Space Between Madness and Brilliance*, who, through the initiative The Icarus Project (now known as the Fireweed Collective) provided the alternative mental health roadmap to my life, evinces, 'I feel like I'm speaking a foreign and clinical language that is useful for navigating my way through the current system but doesn't translate into my own internal vocabulary, where things are so much more fluid and complex.' Contraindications, co-morbidity, transference, autism spectrum, depersonalisation, circumstantiality, abreaction. Some of them have attained the status of mainstream vernacular, each reiteration distilling the last. But more people have this language now. Was she normal or was the world abnormal? Regardless there is no cure. You can talk therapy yourself to death. You can design stop-gap measures (B12, regulate your sleep cycles, decrease alcohol intake, exercise, 'self-care', whatever). You can experiment with a cocktail of substances: a bit of Modafinil here, a little bit of Ritalin there, some Valium or Xanax and cannabis. A nice little piece of psilocybin as a treat. CBD oil is all the rage, at $150 and upwards a pop. You can admit yourself into a psych ward and be looked after by professional care – that is, if you *have* access to health care *and* can afford the best. You can, like the critic Andrea Long Chu, put yourself through something called transcranial magnetic stimulation (TMS), a noninvasive form of brain stimulation where a magnetic field is used to cause an electric current in a specific area of the brain through electromagnetic induction, particularly designed for those with 'treatment-resistant major depressive disorder'. Chu notes that it 'feels like getting flicked in the head by a pencil'. But there is no cure. And with knowledge, as George Scialabba minutely documents in *How To Be Depressed* – through reports written by his multiple therapists and psychiatrists, over decades (1969 to 2016, to be exact) – it is even worse. The mind continually returns to recurring images, past traumas and deep dissatisfactions. Short-term gratifications, such as smooth relations with others and career recognition, help, but are quickly forgotten after the onset of the rush. No different from a drug. Inside the house of depression, the feeling is forever, yet the wretched hope to mitigate its symptoms persist. In the same book, Scialabba publishes a conversation with his friend Christopher Lydon – someone who also 'lives in the neighbourhood of depression' – who remarks, 'Is anything better than a placebo? It's all a kind of fantasy. This is a story without a plot, without characters, without hope, in a way.'

The term 'depression' is so often invoked that it ironically ceases to contain meaning. The Great Depression. The 'meteorological depression'. The lake sits inside a depression. I am so, so, so, so, so depressed! I might need some retail therapy. Some kind of dopamine hit. Memes for the serotonin. These misnomers do not consider the fact that depression is not the opposite of joy; it finds itself inside the wasteland of zero affect. I considered not taking my SSRIs for a week to see if I could write a different essay. But is this disorder more genuine when my neurochemistry isn't blocked by these little pills that purport to alter the shape and texture of my brain? I may still be depressed, but at least I am functioning: for the purposes of conducting conducive relationships with others, for the sake of productivity, for the dream of a so-called fulfilling life. It serves one well to suspend disbelief, and to agree to disagree, with yourself: the exploitation of the sick and ailing by pharmaceutical companies is abhorrent, but these medications are literally making sure some people can live lives, or even continue living at all. Absolutely mad shit. Studies around the brain have been debated and debunked, with new discoveries every few years; no one seems to know exactly what the brain is 'like' – it is a part of us all the time yet it remains an enigma, this formless, sticky mass that works in tandem with everything else. WHAT is the brain? There is no consensus. It's just the brain.

Now, with the cloak of stigma slowly ripped off from its source, everyone is depressed. It may very well be contagious. But are we getting sicker or are we living in an ailing society? In Ann Cvetkovich's *Depression: A Public Feeling*, she maintains that depression is a social problem that is cast as a personal problem, of which factors such as structural inequalities are barely addressed in the literature around it. However, this acknowledgement creates yet another impasse – 'because it's an analysis that frequently admits of no solution'. Cvetkovich continues: 'Saying that capitalism (or colonialism or racism) is the problem does not help me get up in the morning.'

This impasse as a sense of stuckness, which, as Lauren Berlant observes in her essay 'Starved' (2007), is familiar to me. I did not realise I had depression before I learned about the injustices that would result in my terrible home life, but neither did connecting the dots afterwards resolve the malaise. A chicken or the egg question. So what if my mother was insane, affected by decades of intergenerational trauma and the gendered obligations that accompany the grip of patriarchy? So what if my father was also insane, affected by decades of intergenerational trauma that would later lead to alcoholism and other kinds of addictions that would further entrench our impoverished circumstances? We were lucky to live in a rich country. This isn't a call for sympathy (fuck off); rather this is what Berlant calls 'depressive realism', in which they 'do not have the aim of moving beyond *x* but the aim of settling there awhile'. It is a way of not taking on 'optimism's conventional tones'. In other words, if my surrounding environments are already terrible, then why would I deny the attenuating affects that might arise? *Of course* depression is the emotionally appropriate (non)response. The other mental illnesses trail after that like a string of slowly deflating balloons attached to the back of a car. It's perhaps the pressure to seek a resolution that remains the most irrational thing; the fact that checking the fuck out is hardly accepted as a condition of normativity, particularly in the context of capitalist life. The words of fellow depressive Mark Fisher, writing in *Ghosts of My Life*, echo in my head: 'the problem wasn't (just) me, but the culture around me'.

But most nights I finally sleep. That meme comes to mind: 'because it's like being dead without hurting my loved ones'. Away from the keyboard of my brain, ignorant and unaware and at peace. Tomorrow is a dream; she deals with it as it comes. Happiness as an arbitrary demand; a constructed endgame.

Hard Pressed

Grace Tame

The same eyes
that fix on us
were closed before

The same ears
that eavesdrop
were shut before

The hounds
sniffing for blood now
cared not when we were bleeding

All of them
once satisfied by tasteless comments
suddenly hungry for flesh

Signalling absolute feelings
on secondhand stories
they haven't lived

And that's the rub
or lack thereof
a lack of feeling

The unscathed are most scathing
insensitive
or just senseless

How funny it is
that we call them
the press

The untouched
the out of touch
poking and prodding

Demanding we put on a show
but expecting us to pay
expecting us to play, saying

Be the perfect victim
the expert
the counsellor

Tell us about being exploited
while we exploit you
because you are ours

We need you
we own you
you are sensational

Suicide Dogs

David Stavanger

1.
There is a bridge in Scotland where over fifty dogs
have inexplicably leapt to their deaths, plummeting
from parapet past green stone. Many believe it to be
possessed by the devil. Others claim the dogs are lost
in the pursuit of wild mink and tear off into mid-air,
keening for game. There have been reports of some
surviving their brush with death, only to return for a
second shot. These dogs understand what is at stake,
such leaps premeditated attempts to be closer to us
in every conceivable way.

2.
Dogs don't need to be taught how to smell.
They do need to be taught where to sniff –
along the seams of self-harm, underneath
a sudden calm where tense vapours settle.
Their nostrils can be trained to pick up poison
or the scent of gas, ears pin pricked for the sudden
ignition of an oven outside normal hours of use.
Suicide dogs begin building their own vocabulary
of suspicious odours, working out that ideation
will find nostrils quicker than food. Strictly speaking,
the dog smells intent. Trainers say these dogs know
when people are thinking of leaving through body cues,
electrical signals and other ways not yet named. Perhaps
a quietening of the voice. A loudening thought. Forgoing sleep.
Drastic changes in behaviour, such as laughter or cleaning up a room,
result in the dogs exhibiting attention-getting behaviours:
whining, pawing, or anxious barking. Some people try
and write a final note to their companion, which these dogs
quickly intercept, licking hands until a pen is placed down.

3.
There are signs. A dog jumping a fence forces you
to go outside and interact with the world. If it lays at your feet,
they have registered the absence of a smile. Becoming less
concerned about personal appearance, a dog will excessively
groom itself. They recognise the shapes of fragile –
slumped over, static, responding to a lack of fear
with bowed head and tucked tail. Research shows that dogs
don't know what tears are. They do know they assist in
detecting despair on a loved one's breath, a change in mood
triggered by the slightest tremor of the lower lip.

4.
Dogs can be trained to stay with the person during an attempt
or to press a phone's emergency button with a paw. Part
alarm clock, part smoke detector. Other dogs fail to go for help.
A suicide dog will bite a stranger up the road in exchange
for the authorities being contacted, never reluctant to seek
professional help. Some have appeared as willing witness
at a coronial inquest. Others have identified their owner's remains,
refusing to leave the side of those they were sent to protect.
They will never abandon you. They will forever hold
the slender bone of hope, tender in their jaws.

5.
Initial outcomes are encouraging. It has been found
that gun dogs are better than hunting hounds; earth dogs
tune into latent wishes; sled dogs follow a figure favouring
a fast exit. Such dogs will howl if sharp objects start calling out.
Cliffs are avoided on long walks. Once vehicles are present,
they examine exhaust pipes for trace isolation. One dog lay
on a passenger seat, refusing to exit until the car was impounded.
The handler informed the news channel this is a 'death reaction',
indicating a high chance that a body will be found in the vehicle
if left in its garage for another day.

6.
Surveying a room for rafters or the height of a doorway,
barking and scratching apparent warnings against high risk activities
like taking baths, climbing chairs, or staring out to sea.
A negative view of the self requires the dog to lie still
on the threshold, one ear up in case their owner says
'If I wasn't here, would you miss me?'
When this animal chooses not to sleep beside you
it is a sure sign for distant relatives to come close.
No one can prove conclusively what suicide dogs are thinking.
They are not yet able to make funeral arrangements.
While they note the giving away of clothes and books,
they reserve judgement as far as one can tell, pretending
to be pinned beneath furniture before it is taken.

7.
Scientists say there are no guarantees.
Not every suicide is preventable.
Success can't be dissected in post-mortem reports.
The number of dogs with this ability is unknown,
shining a small torch into a pack of eyes.
Scientists are certain these canines are born
with an innate sense of our purpose, our light.

They will not bury the evidence that we exist.

Panic in the time of Covid-19

Anna Spargo-Ryan

Late 2021, Melbourne. Like many people, I have been sitting in my house for months or years or eternity, venturing out only to see my parents at a distance and buy enough chocolate to get me through. Unlike many people, this is really very similar to what I was already doing.

It feels obscene to have an anxiety disorder during a pandemic. At the time of writing, more than five million people have died. It seems vile to look at the news, social media, even out the window, and think, 'I'm afraid'. Everyone is afraid. The experience of being anxious suddenly feels both universal and individualistic.

I keep thinking about what it might be like to rock up at a hospital right now for mental illness reasons. Not imminent real danger, but the step before that, the not being able to cope. I imagine a triage nurse saying, 'What's the matter?' and me saying, 'I feel really anxious.' And they would go, 'What do you mean?' and I would explain how the world feels like it's caving in, that things seem far away, that my heart won't stop racing, that my head is going to pop off. What could they say except, 'Everyone does' and 'Please leave'?

What is the place for mental illness in global chaos?

I started dwelling on this in December of 2019. It had been hot for so many days in a row. The ground was tinder, kindling. Dry brush, trees reaching for a spark. Thick smoke travelled hundreds of kilometres to blanket disconnected cities. On the news, people from a small Victorian town sought safety from the flames on their local beach. Fire was near and it blocked the sun. They cowered in a red darkness. An authority told them that when things got really bad, a whistle would sound, and they would have to get in the water.

I thought, 'Those people are brave.'

I thought, 'I couldn't do that.'

And then after that I thought, 'I'm a danger to others.'

I made a sort of 'bushfire plan', the way they tell you to. *What will you do in a fire?* If the fires did come to my largely safe suburban house – very unlikely, though sometimes the park at the end of the street gets lit up – there would not be time for my hesitation or paranoia. I would have to sit with my fears and wait for the flames to come and I could not, for even one moment, ask someone I loved to wait there with me. To please hold on a second and breathe the black air while I tried to undo a lifetime of disordered thinking. I am a liability, an obstacle, the last person you want in your zombie apocalypse squad. So, I decided, I would probably die in my burnt-down house, hoping my family had made it to safety, and that would be the correct thing to happen.

At the beginning of the Covid-19 isolation – especially in Australia, where the risk was comparatively low, before Melbourne went into its hectic and repeated lockdowns – many of us were buoyed by the urgency and the novelty (such is the nature of our enormous privilege). Every day there was something new to watch or learn or participate in. I went to viewing parties and friends' birthdays. I rocked up at a dozen book launches; for the first, I washed my hair and used concealer, but by the sixth I didn't even apologise for my stringy, grimy appearance. That was around the time my daughter pushed a hole clean through her pyjamas – she had been wearing them for fifteen days straight.

In the beginning, the experience of fear did feel universal. Something I had held for my whole life became an emotion for everyone. People who had always felt secure were thrust into unease.

As general society shifted into digital spaces, everything that had been withheld from me was possible. Now that the public needed connection, years of technological obstacles and red tape disintegrated. Writers' festivals I had longed for were in my living room. Broadway shows, museums, concerts. Even having a coffee (or a Milo) with faraway family was possible. Almost everyone worked from home. Almost everyone went outside with trepidation. Almost every single person in the country – the world – suddenly had similar access needs to me. The way I existed, which was largely in my extremely localised safe space / living room, rapidly became ordinary.

It's hard to explain what this meant. Whole humiliating interactions were lifted. I no longer had to justify myself when I asked for leniency on Travelling Places and Going Far. I was asked to do a couple of media appearances, and I said 'yes' without offering contingencies about probably not being able to get into the studio but I would really try.

Other people apologised to *me* for not being able to meet me in person. I spent breathtaking moments on the other side of the most difficult conversations I had ever had.

'This is it,' I thought. 'People will understand my experience now.'

I was, trapped in my house as always, suddenly a viable human again.

As it is for so many living with serious mental illness, a good portion of my life is occupied with trying to explain why something isn't possible. Anxiety is widely acknowledged and less stigmatised than it once was, but a combination of fear (both rational and clinically significant) and self-loathing means skirting the truth. Sorry I can't make it, I'm ill – true, but I'll tell you it's food poisoning because panic disorder is gross.

At the start of the first lockdown, I was buoyed by spare energy not expended on making excuses. There were no plans I had to cancel, no meetings I needed to move. I no longer had to practise a breezy, 'Shall we just do this one over the phone?' as though it were perfectly sound logic and not a side effect of my heart trying to thunder its way out of my chest. I signed up for everything, bought all the tickets I could find. I did online courses and attended virtual lectures. I wrote about what it was like in Melbourne in the thick isolated winter, without the usual comforts of footy and open fires at the pub, and people read them and sighed that they, too, felt worried and uncertain. Like I did.

Faced with the prospect of millions of anxious and depressed Australians, state and federal governments took (small) tangible steps to supporting mental health. Mental health care plans were bumped from ten subsidised sessions to twenty. JobKeeper and increased JobSeeker payments allowed people to keep the lights on, put food on the table, and access health care, all basic human rights that provide a better foundation for mental wellbeing. There was, amid the realisation of a lifetime's panic 'for no reason', a small mental illness utopia. Not happiness, just an equalisation.

Until there wasn't. By the second and third and fourth Melbourne lockdowns, an interesting thing occurred which was this: disability, once again, was absorbed by More Pressing Concerns. We weren't all simply working from home, but working and living in one confined space during the apocalypse. The noise my mental illnesses usually make – shrieking for someone to please lay all their body weight on top of me – were drowned out by a population of people experiencing the same feelings for the first time. My panic is chronic and blunt; theirs was newly urgent. It sucked oxygen like a flame.

Over the course of months, my mental health deteriorated. It wasn't only the remote learning with two miserable teenagers, or the deadlines that couldn't be moved even at the end of the world, or never having one moment of time alone. In an abled-centric hellscape, where swathes of people had suddenly become cognisant of what it might be like to face access issues or chronic pain or illness, those of us who had always known evaporated.

At some point, during a lockdown that has blended into all the others, I went to bed and stayed there for nearly 72 hours. My bones felt like they had been filled with mercury. No one knew; blurring the Zoom background meant every meeting looked the same.

During these lockdown periods, disabled people and advocates shouted at length about what things could look like when the danger had passed. Covid had eliminated so much red tape – services and payments always deemed 'too hard' had quickly become available, when the right kind of people needed them. What if, the disability community asked, that kind of accessibility could continue? What if it could be formalised, written into policy, made part of every employment contract?

Not to spoil it for the optimistic among us, but it didn't. As vaccination numbers went up, people went back to work and school and...forgot. They caught trains and drove cars to locations still out of reach for many disabled people, like me. Hesitantly, sure, but without obstacle.

When I happily offered Zoom meetings, which had been convenient – necessary – for almost two years, they frowned instead. They said, 'Ugh, haven't we had enough of those?' They said, 'It's time to open up!'

'Oh, right,' I said, nodding in my digital frame. 'Yes, of course,' I agreed, thinking of the handful of local shops that feel safe for me to visit.

'Let us see our friends!' they said, and I reflected on how I had seen more of my friends during Covid than I had in the decade before;

that I had been able to support them remotely instead of letting them down; that I had shown up for them, in these virtual spaces.

I sat at my desk in my living room, where I have always sat, and opened up. I put on my good jeans. I sent emails from the pocket of safety I've spent years creating. And I grieved for that isolation period, when I could be alone on the outside, too.

Bad Dog Moon Fever

Samson J. L. Soulsby

Madness runs in my family
like greyhounds,
over-fast skeletons with wild eyes and a fear of fireworks
sprinting towards early graves,
not knowing how to get off the track
so it goes around another generation with its teeth out
ready to take a bite of you if you're too slow,

which you are.

You start waking up in the night pulling teeth
out of your head from where your brain
chews on itself.
You start playing fetch with your demons
every solitary walk, hoping this time
they don't remember the way home,

but they do.

There's bad dogs under your skin
and every night is a full moon;
there's bad dogs fighting
to hold onto your bones
just to bury them when no-one is looking,

and no-one is ever looking.
There's a wretched howling inside:
it gets louder and louder
every time it hears itself echo

because it's lonely

but can't be trusted in company.
There is something deep and mean
in a dog too hungry for too long
on a chain too short,
bristled, hackles up, all sharp shapes,
half-expecting a beating,
half-awaiting the hand it feeds on
to come back for more,
and beg to be bitten
again.

Some curses are contagious
only in the blood,
passed down like a riddle—
what can you give away and still have?

brought out from dark marrow
by the fever-bright moon,

itself some heavenly magnifying glass,
burning you up with second-hand sunlight,
the fascination of wanting desperately
to understand
why,

until your life and the countless others before you
here and gone
are vivisected,
scrutinised,
and, still,
inexplicable.

At best, it's a halfway shifting thing
wearing your skin,
hoping not to be seen
in the light of day,

by chance wise enough to live
with the window open

to let out the howl

and let in the stars.

ODE TO BAD MEDICINE

Brooke Scobie

When wallaby slows to listen
There grows bad medicine
Fires suffocate and fill the air with felted grey
Desert birds fall from the sky
Flesh dripping from their softened bones
There grows bad medicine

Lavender glory smothers Grandma's hands
Trust is built on stolen lands
Bridges are swallowed into earth
Magpie's voice falls silent
There grows bad medicine

Where whispers scream and water burns
No one picks up the phone
Atmosphere thicker than mucous
When echidna's quills curl under
There grows bad medicine

Wallflowers and Evergreens

Kirli Saunders

I count the threads in the rug
on my psychologist's floor

gaze lowered
eye contact avoidant

this is how I find feathers
but don't see the spirits
that leave them

she tells me
rage's underbelly
is *grief*

I imagine thumbing
sacred geometry –
fronds soft in palms
toes   s e p a r a t e d
by summered grass
and bark peels

the eucalyptus
staining the air blue
where the hues
of beauty

are seen through tears
and this
elation and depth
are welcomed   simultaneously

                                    I return to sterility
                                         and wonder
               how to be (held)
                                                  in spaces
                                    devoid of seasons

                                         where time is measured by
                         clockface
                         and replaces
          eucalyptus blooming
               echidna trains
                    winds that change
                    moon who wanes

                                              I think rage
                                    must be manufactured
                                    in the same place as
                                         plastic plants

     with the willingness to wilt
                    withdrawn

     softness
                    starched and sewn

     fragility
               propped up
                    by falsity

                    for appearances

                                    I imagine us
                                    fabricating ourselves
                                              to be
                                         in the world

all wallflowers and evergreens

I realise
I trust more deeply
in the tree
that releases
its seeds
after it
burns

Elegy for a (Hated) Body

Sara M. Saleh

How many fingers does it take to do what
I never thought I would do to this body?

Dust shelves, fold sheets, then shove a fist
back of the throat to bring order to my body.

On Friday nights I don't sing, I hurtle towards the
Hate, the sink, this is the only way to accept this body.

An unholy ritual and I am a stranger,
I cup the ashes, the impurities of somebody.

I pull and pinch and stretch and scab
to be touched just enough by anybody.

They slip hips on as costume now, and I use
a knife to cut, to make room for more body.

Page after page, I learn my Devil so I learn
my God, but can either exist out-of-body?

Dr Diaz says, *the rot is deep, but you are not an
unspectacular thing.*
Lover says, *I am tired of carrying this whole body.*

Don't die, the ancestors say but they did not
prepare me for when I betray and call it body.

All these years, I still don't know how
to say 'forgive me',
I am an elegy before I am a body.

Runtime

Omar Sakr

One episode in I declare *I would die for them*. Any character from my life is worth dying for when they're on a screen. *It's so easy* to love them there. I want Tia Kofi to rip-start a chainsaw in my heart *I swear* this sandwich is so good *kill me*. We're dancing in a flood of light and *my body won't stop* trying to find another way to close. Like any failed alchemist *all I know is how* to take a good thing and make of it a menace. This is what the world did with God & yes *I am the world* & *no*, I won't learn my lessons. I'm in the metaphor factory again fighting for my beard *to be* a beard and on the way out this jalabiya becomes my eternal shroud. No, song. Today I'm going to run at the *police* barricades in a lip sync for my life. I'm tired of mouthing what I must in order to survive. I'm going to run at the gun after I kiss a faggot on the lips. I am the faggot on my lips and I am running toward a choice that *is not inevitable*. Doom feels so delicious on my skin. Don't you love to shiver in the ending, isn't it in the ending that we get *to triumph*, or is that only after tragedy? In the after or before, *tell me* what's waiting, is it a gun or parade? I'm trying to cook up a revolution here, *of course* the kitchen's on fire. I can put it out or read the secret songs of smoke, but not both. I'm reading *the earth* with a sore melodious throat, watching the house sashay away to great acclaim in a little black dress. It *was never* my house, never my mind, never *mine*, but I own this dress *believe* me, I want to tear out *the good pages of every book* and eat the cheap paper. The good pages will be those I land on, or the ones without people. *Fuck*, I think I finally understand the Romantics—& this is why I *laugh* stumbling hysterical free as I run & *run* toward the only certainty I know.

The Queue

Rebecca Rushbrook

I am standing in line
to petition for somewhere to live.
Thirty-six of us, socially distanced,
uneasy as we meet each other's eyes.
There is one house.

With her mascara and curls,
the real estate girl
is more Disney than Dickensian.
But here I approach,
an Oliver Twist,
clutching my application
like an empty bowl
I have no right to fill.

I have three children.
I have a dog, a job,
a washing machine…
Yesterday I was 'normal'.
Packing the lunches
and finding the uniforms,
sculling coffee,
and shouting too loudly
as I hurried us all out the door
in time for our day.

Then the floor fell away.
Our rental is selling.
Now I wake every morning
in a burning building
and it's money, not water

that will put out this fire
and I don't have enough.

So I line up
with my single income
and the weight of my family
heavy in my chest.
The real estate girl
smiles at two tradies.
I look at them and think,
'Two paychecks, no kids',
I look at the application
and wonder
how hard it would be
to hide our dog.

He's a Labrador
with bad back legs.
He is the heart of my daughter.

I thought I could carry us.
When the marriage that made them
hit its iceberg and sank,
I collected the flotsam
and built us a boat.
Learned to sail by myself.
I was getting the hang of it.
Keeping one hand on the rudder.
Fishing with my foot for our dinner.
But these waves were made for liners
and my craft is too flimsy.
This water pours into it
faster than I can bail.

You'll have seen them,
the polar bears
in open ocean,

nudging their cubs
to keep them together,
as they desperately scan
for any land that will hold them.

The rentals have melted.
The lenders won't loan.
Paying your way
doesn't earn you a home.
I am lining up
with thirty-six people
clutching white knuckled
to the edge of this crack
we are sliding through.

Far over our heads,
the currawongs sail
their clear paths
to their nests by the river.
My eyes ride on their trajectories.
There are tents in the bush down there.
More every week.

At the psychiatrist's office seeking hormones like a thirsty snail seeking water, soft and gooey but hiding my insides

Anne Rachael Ross

motel room sorta carpets
window to brick alley
I sit across from him
sorta sipping tepid water
he doesn't drink any
scratches on a pad
I have three days of expired prescription hormones at home
have been waiting for this appointment for three weeks
(In the UK people wait three years, don't we have it good)
          '…Childhood friends?'
How to explain too many female friends equalled fag at school
how I have those friends now anyway
      'I mean, I did play with my cousins a lot'
Well fit together teleology of realisation, repression, acceptance to
  now
sip water
        it's all reverse causality
like reading trans into my Pluto Sagittarius
but less affirming, more con
firming some square he ticks
the clock ticks I sip water
questions tip into awkward
'If you could have a vagina'
he asks me
      sip water
think of why I haven't thought about it
say something about $30,000
and no parents' private

or patience with the changes
I'm only starting now
or—
                    'No' he says
'If I had a magic button you could push'
I think my Yes was more to push
the very real enter-key to send the letter
to let me dodge the draft of manhood
as a medically designated faggot
I sip water, dip my head as
he says 'You have very fine features,
              and have a lot to work with'
A body shaped well for his ideal
object of transsexual
this may be an unfair reading
but doctor – read the room
                    it's history
when this was the only question asked
and Drs simply asked themselves   (so don't *we* have it good)
        but this heavy unthunk of the unlimits
I'd've done for his pen stroke on a letter hangs
the sort of thought that sticks in your throat
no matter how much water you swallow
all pride, smile, 'thank you' to the compliment
his frames catch the fluorescence
I unclench my glass
he   '…can recommend trial of hormone replacement therapy'
smiling like he doesn't really believe in the gate he's keeping
        I've sincerely had it good
but I apologise
like any anachronistic *it* I've had good
has to do with the sunlight
by the ocean last Sunday
        months later
hopping between rock pools
brilliant post-swim almonds
bursting between molars

as we lay on towels in the sand
quoting Anakin Skywalker at each other
letting the water seep from my hair into my towel
nothing to do with a doctor
and his creepy checklist

The Birth of Judas

Paris Rosemont

The catch with the transformative
Is that you cannot rewind the clock
Pandora's box unleashed
Gives birth
To a fresh brand of hell

From virgin to damaged goods
Forevermore
Even if you are born again
Your hymen
Might have a thing or two
To say about that

Curious thing, the birthing experience
Simultaneously, two beings are born
Child and mother
Intertwined

What then is a childless mother?
Still a mother
Though incomplete
Her life's purpose
Stillborn
Would that the beating of her heart
Find stillness too

Nay, she was born to suffer
Dripping chunks of flesh
From her wounded heart
Haemorrhaging
A slow, painful limp towards death

Gaping holes
In the shadow board
Of where her little loves used to be
If you look closely
You may observe the outlines
Of murderous tools
That were used as weapons
By a hand that once loved her

Permission to forget

Lillian Rodrigues-Pang

You   have permission to forget
You   do not need to hold on
You   do not need to know

Thorazine   Perphenazine   Clozapine   Asenapine   Cariprazine
The prazoles and the dones
Melt from mind and tongue

I no longer need to know
No knowing
Not to know
Not to go
Get repeats
Blood tests
Trials
Checks

I take my permission
I forget
I wipe clean
I pour water not to sip with meds but to cleanse
From veins   as all   cascade away
Waterfalls of memories

A deluge smashing solid ground
I crumble seeing your stiff form
Death
Your laughter   your love   your soul   becomes water
Flows through sediment
Away
Filtering to a realm I cannot follow

My heaving heart
My struggle to breathe
The sound of realities colliding
When you and I were truly in the one room
In stillness
In loss
Your body decaying
Enzymes doing their transformative work
My mind deconstructing
This story
This event
Your touch, so cold, to a hug, a pause, a goodbye

The important work of erasing
Useless   names of medications
Useless   words in argument
Useless   hopes that were held close to my heart
Nurtured in my dreams

I allow the decomposition of recall
I purposefully forget
Defiantly letting go of medical details
Names   quantities   colours   days taken   or forgotten
No more judgement
No more measuring

I choose to forget the way that your eyes became a tool
Red, scared, loose, away, with me, volatile, safe, drained, angry
Seeing me, not seeing me, laughing, secretive, judgemental

I choose to forget that I quantified you
on the nanosecond of approach
I assessed your mood
Your meds were just one measure
My fear a far greater one

Magic Numbers

Ariel Riveros Pavez

A situated scene: People throw numbers out there like numbers are dice. You could be ungenerous about that and say it's magical thinking. But magical thinking has its own virtues if it's a practice. Magicians and scientists both share laboratory. Magic is pre-modern and so is religion and both had solutions via practice in their day. Christianity picked on magic. The rest is situated history. Dawkins claims magical realism for his science but more in the Carl Sagan way where your mouth is open in a meme. The cachet of literature for Dawkins oooooh such Oxbridge emperor stuff. Throwing numbers like dice is just casting a spell. Some numbers are kinda random others though are referenced. The numbers mean things beyond an internally consistent symbol for quantity and measurement. The references go back to numerology and whatever that Platonic looking Chaldean numbers Google ad is. And all that the one, like a unitary Pythagorean monad, the monad of whatever-(ything)-it-is, and the window closes. My apartment is the camera. I got a good image of the view. I don't know why people don't throw out numbers to each other in bars more often and not just staff. Referential number throwing gets my interest. It's a chance for a story when I ask them what they mean. Especially without involving the internet content about it. The referential number is a gambit for a personal truth because cachet of math. It's so 3487.

Bag of Feathers

Tess Ridgway

Stories about psychosis are like telling someone your dreams
the little chiming significances only crash down on my own head
as a maraca did during music therapy back in the loony bin

To other people it's like I've emptied a bag of feathers
over their heads – the specifics spill and spook, white ghosts
they fan out – never quite landing

It's like drug stories (& are drug stories the new war stories?)
they only make sense housed in their own box
like broken odds & ends

Back in the shadow days
when I piggy backed on the sun & leaped to the moon without rest
I wore a new world like a crown & lengthened my spine to fill it out
I forced ends to meet like making two snakes kiss

Two years on, the memories fly in like fat slow flies, I bat them away
that time is a mound of mud I try to pat into a vase
though a few things I know for sure:

It began at Mermaid Pools when I slid down a waterfall & hit the
    shallows
I overextended my knee & tore a ligament but kept moving
& after the doctor equipped me with a knee brace
black Velcro-strapped, I continued to grind down my gears
pedalling up hills & swanning through parties

The pain wore on & I propped myself up in cafe corners
skolling cappuccinos & chewing codeine
& I started to count broken knees that matched my own

I'd clamped onto a pattern & I kept pulling on that gold tooth to seize
    my bounty

I played my records in reverse & tuned my radio just right
& it only made me speed up before it slowed me down
like the climax to 2001: A Space Odyssey
it looned around my head like a clump of midges

I had two baths: one with torn tea bags & bit-open propolis capsules
a squid ink, leafy brew I stewed in easy listening to Smooth FM
(all the love songs were dedicated to me!)

The other I had outside under the night's sky
in low-light black&white I plucked slugs
from under the lip of the bath and laid them on my face
with the night draped over us we softened up to each other

The night pre-hospital my sister took me to bed
she held my arm tight & stuck her nails in my arms to keep me down
and (though I can't prove it) jabbed me with a needle
to let me sleep (let me die) *am I going to die?* I sobbed exhausted
(I was sure there was a silver bullet in my brain, a tumour – but I
    can't prove it)

Next morning in the hospital waiting room, I cracked
white Styrofoam cups over my chest
the earth's contours compressed and bled magma
it felt cool on my chest

I had quit sleep & it let me see what I wanted to see
because maybe I was royalty or the writer of M*A*S*H.
The world was Play Doh & I ate it without shame
I was balanced on a precipice like cutting a ruby red grapefruit
& tonguing the knife-edge juice

It was all a gas & I was fine, I explained to the doctor
I'm conducting 3 orchestras at once
I was reaching a crescendo, I was butting my head against the ceiling
like a loaded broom handle –
I was going to hoist myself on the sky's shoulders & lick the sun
I could taste it – a two-dollar coin dipped in melted butter –
this prize pig was gonna fly

Dad, am I a genius?
'You're very smart, darling.'

Under The Influence

Michelle Rickerby

There was that time they found you
hiding in the pantry.
                            Wearing nothing
but a pair of Woolies sheer control tights,
                                    swatting at the bubbles you said
            were sent to spy on you.

when it feels heavy

Bhenji Ra

(when it feels heavy)
do not abandon yourself,
feel the weight of your body –
all of its edges and sides
hold every part / kiss every part
like a friend, newborn, lover
remember
all that supports you
is in you.

Flesh
Hope One

High pitched screams
Palm connecting to cheek
The weight of an adult body
Hitting the wall

Wailing,
Pukana eyes
Stiff lips
Moustache hair curved over the top
Like a fringe
Nostrils widened
Chest puffed
Clenched fists

Does he think she's a man?
His actions are telling me so
45kg woman
Who would never hurt a soul

Scars decorate his back
From the pulling of a metal coat hanger
Dragging its way through the mud
Through flesh, through blood
Through a young boy's love

The foster care system did its job
To create an unhealed
Highly aggressive
Maori man

Under the bed she lay
Face down
Ears tightly clenched by the palm of her hand
The pressure enough to create a dip
Lalalalalala she sings
Over filtered sounds of mayhem

The thumps soon became subwoofers at 18
Smashing plates soon became sound effects
Adding to the repertoire of beats she's creating
Hi hats to match the cold blood of a snake
He bites her in silence
Venom fills her veins
Plunging fire

These are the stories of their daughters
The damage haunts
Floats like smog
Clouded visions
Of poison

CARRY ALL MY HURT AWAY

Steven Oliver

VERSE 1
I CLOSE MY EYES, TAKE A BREATH AND I COUNT TO THREE
I'M TRYING TO REACQUAINT MYSELF WITH MY IDENTITY
I'M TRYING TO FIGURE OUT, REMEMBER WHO'S INSIDE THE
    SHELL
YOU'D THINK I'D KNOW ME OH SO WELL
BUT LATELY OTHER PEOPLE WANNA
TELL ME WHO I AM AND WHO I GOT TO BE
STRANGERS, FRIENDS, PEERS, COLLEAGUES EVEN FAMILY
SAYING I GOTTA BE THIS, I GOTTA BE THAT
I GOTTA TELL JOKES, I GOTTA SPEAK FACTS
I GOT TO BE WHATEVER THEY NEED, JUST DON'T BE WHO I
    NEED FOR ME
JUST SIMPLY USE THE NAME, JUST SIMPLY USE THE FAME
JUST SIMPLY PLAY THE GAME AND SIMPLY STAY THE SAME
BUT LATELY SIMPLE SITUATIONS HAVE ME FEELING USED
THEY WANNA HAVE MY BEING BUT DISPOSE OF MY TRUTH
COS IF I TELL THEM THAT I'M FEELING SAD, THAT I'M FEELING
    DOWN
THEY IGNORE THE HURT THAT'S IN MY WORDS BECAUSE THEY
    WANT THE CLOWN
AND SO, I DON THE MASK, PERFORMING THE TASK, I'M GIVING
    THEM WHAT THEY ASK
BUT I'LL NEVER LAST IF I CAN'T GET THE PAIN TO PASS

CHORUS
MY MIND IS SAYING THAT THE PAIN WILL NEVER GO AWAY
MY HEART IS SAYING THAT IT MIGHT'NT MAKE IT THROUGH
    THE DAY
MY SOUL IS SAYING DON'T YOU LISTEN TO A WORD THEY SAY

TAKE YOUR SPIRIT AND YOUR BEING AND LIVE TO FIGHT
   ANOTHER DAY
MY MIND IS SAYING THAT THE PAIN WILL NEVER GO AWAY
MY HEART IS SAYING THAT IT MIGHT'NT MAKE IT THROUGH
   THE DAY
MY SOUL IS SAYING DON'T YOU LISTEN TO A WORD THEY SAY
TAKE YOUR SPIRIT AND YOUR BEING AND LIVE TO FIGHT
   ANOTHER DAY

VERSE 2
I'M SEEKING SILENCE NOW
I'M HIDING IN A ROOM, DON'T WANNA STAND OUT IN A CROWD
ANXIETY IS TAMING ME AS PEOPLE GET TO BLAMING ME
THAT I GOT WHAT I DESERVED BECAUSE I WANTED TO BE
   HEARD
SO NOW, I'M LOSING CONTROL AND THOUGH I KNOW THAT
   LOVE DON'T JUDGE ME
THERE ARE THINGS I WITHHOLD
BECAUSE THE SHAME I PUT UPON MYSELF WHAT I'M GOING
   THROUGH
MAKES ME FEEL THAT I'M NO LONGER THE PERSON PEOPLE
   ONCE KNEW
I TELL MYSELF THAT I'M A LIE, I'M NOT EVEN SOME GUY
I'M JUST A SOULLESS TALKING SHADOW IN THE DARK
   WALKING BLIND
FORGETTING WHO I AM JUST TO GET THROUGH MY DAY
BUT IF I DON'T CONFRONT MYSELF THEN THE PAIN ONLY STAYS
AND I WANNA SHARE MY HURT BUT I GET BLAMED FOR THE
   FAME
SO, WHAT IF I SPEAK MY TRUTH AND IT'S EXACTLY THE SAME
BUT IN THE END I NEED TO REALISE MY LIFE IS FOR ME
AND IF I LET THEIR JUDGEMENT CAGE ME, I'LL NEVER BE FREE

CHORUS
MY MIND IS SAYING THAT THE PAIN HAS GOT TO GO AWAY
MY HEART IS SAYING THAT IT'S GOT TO MAKE IT THROUGH THE
   DAY

MY SOUL IS SAYING THAT I'VE STILL GOT SO MUCH LEFT TO SAY
TAKE MY SPIRIT AND MY BEING AND LIVE TO FIGHT ANOTHER
   DAY
MY MIND IS SAYING THAT THE PAIN HAS GOT TO GO AWAY
MY HEART IS SAYING THAT IT'S GOT TO MAKE IT THROUGH THE
   DAY
MY SOUL IS SAYING THAT I'VE STILL GOT SO MUCH LEFT TO SAY
TAKE MY SPIRIT AND MY BEING AND LIVE TO FIGHT ANOTHER
   DAY

BRIDGE
WITHIN MY CHAOS I FOUND MY CLARITY
AND IN MY LIKENESS DID LEARN DISPARITY
IN ABUNDANT WASTE DID I SEEK MY NEED
COS ONLY BEING CAGED MADE ME UNDERSTAND FREE
WITHIN MY CHAOS I FOUND MY CLARITY
AND IN MY LIKENESS DID LEARN DISPARITY
IN ABUNDANT WASTE DID I SEEK MY NEED
COS ONLY BEING CAGED MADE ME UNDERSTAND FREE

CHORUS
MY MIND IS SAYING THAT THE PAIN IS GONNA GO AWAY
MY HEART IS SAYING EVERYTHING IS GONNA BE OKAY
MY SOUL IS SAYING THAT I'VE STILL GOT SO MUCH LEFT TO SAY
TAKE MY SPIRIT AND MY BEING AND LIVE TO FIGHT ANOTHER
   DAY
MY MIND IS SAYING THAT THE PAIN IS GONNA GO AWAY
MY HEART IS SAYING EVERYTHING IS GONNA BE OKAY
MY SOUL IS SAYING THAT I'VE STILL GOT SO MUCH LEFT TO SAY
TAKE MY SPIRIT, WATCH IT SOAR AND CARRY ALL MY HURT
   AWAY

OUTRO
WITHIN MY CHAOS I FOUND MY CLARITY
AND IN MY LIKENESS DID LEARN DISPARITY
IN ABUNDANT WASTE DID I SEEK MY NEED
COS ONLY BEING CAGED MADE ME UNDERSTAND FREE

WITHIN MY CHAOS I FOUND MY CLARITY
AND IN MY LIKENESS DID LEARN DISPARITY
IN ABUNDANT WASTE DID I SEEK MY NEED
COS ONLY BEING CAGED MADE ME UNDERSTAND FREE

Discount Superman

Nat's What I Reckon

When I was a kid I always thought that being a superhero was the way to go. I'll shoot for that – it probably pays well, everyone's in great shape, and when presented with any distress, you can just fuck off, get changed and fucken deal with it, you know? It's great. I'll become a 'super' man.

Solid call, I reckon, even at that age. Maybe I should have taken that info with me to my job placement meetings when I was on the dole. Don't think they would have appreciated that, to be honest. I definitely did score some fucken shit jobs along the way and they definitely weren't being any kind of superhero.

What I did end up with was a laundry list of mental health problems, which is seemingly kind of the opposite of superpowers at first glance. When presented with a load of distress, I usually just stay in the same clothes and have a massively unimpressive meltdown.

I grew up in a fundamentalist Christian church. I was born into it. Straight out of the gates, no time to waste. As I was learning to eat, walk and other useful life shit, I was also taught to believe in God. That was the routine for a while. My dad was a minister and my mum was a singer in the church. It was very involved, a full-time thing. I would go to church several times a Sunday and lots of other church things during the week. I did the rough maths, and if you were someone who goes to church once a week, I reckon I had gone more fucken times by the age of 16 than most people would have in their whole lives...about 60+ years worth of church.

That routine didn't really work out that well for me, unfortunately, with the church.

Eventually Dad left the church and my family split, and that was a really fucken tough time. I missed my dad a lot and didn't really have anyone to talk to about what the fuck was going on for me.

If you talk to people about what's going on for you at church they often tell you to turn to your bible, you know? Which is fine, if that works for you, but I'm a fucked up eight-year-old missing my dad and not doing well in other parts of my life either. I was in tears all the time, suffering huge amounts of heartache and fear daily. I didn't really know what to do with all that stuff at that age...so I just began collecting mental health problems like they were fucken baseball cards. I thought I had the whole set for a minute. Not sure it's worth much?

But there was a lot of that – a lot of 'turning to God' – and it wasn't really helping.

I eventually left the church and continued to suffer a great deal. I was kind of a fuckup of a kid that grew up to be a bit of a fuckup too, but I did grow up understanding what a tricky head looks like.

I didn't really end up with those superpowers, but I ended up doing other stuff with this distress that my head puts me through. It's not super romantic, but my way of coping is to take the piss – that's my thing. You find the space that you're in, you find where the walls are by taking the piss. There's fuck-all I can do about feeling uncomfortable and anxious, so I may as well have a laugh at some shit around me and lighten the mood a little.

It's not at first glance a superpower, being able to take the piss. SUPER TAKE-THE-PISS MAN...it's probably not going to get picked up by Marvel at any point – I wonder what special ability they have? Just flies in, tells you that 'your finger-toed shoes and fedora make ya look like you're maybe trying to look a little too laid back' and then just take off?

It's not something I have known what to do with for most of my life, my mental health problems. I've seen a lot of people about it, taken a lot of medications, fucked up a bunch. It's not cheap therapy either. Fuck, you can drop some serious coin on self-care, but it's worth it, you've gotta keep working on it. Your mental health is a bit like an old clapped out RX7, kinda keeps shitting the gear, it uses a lot of fuel, makes a lot of noise and it breaks down a lot...Fun to drive when it's running properly but for the most part it's gonna fucken take a bit of work to keep on the road.

You've gotta do something with all this noisy head shit. I'm lucky enough to be pretty fucking useless at everything else that all I can do is be creative and take the piss, so that's what I do. I'm strangely lucky that my anxious and occasionally depressed outlook on the world has found me a job cracking jokes about it all.

I tell ya what, every day is a fucken bit of work for me, but it makes me who I am, whether I fucken like it or not.

It helps me understand parts of the world in different ways and that's not always a bad thing. If I've got a mate who's in distress, I may not be fucken Superman, but if they say to me, 'Fuck, I've had a shit day, everything and everyone can get fucked', or maybe they're just crying...I ask 'What's going on?' And they say, 'I dunno...?'

...In that moment, I kinda know.

In that minute I kind of am a superman of sorts.

I kinda get it, I don't know how to fix it, but I see ya in that moment and I give a shit.

I wouldn't give all this tricky shit up for missing out on being able to understand people I care about.

It's always worth it, always worth the work.

It's all worth it to be able to love ya mates a bit more.

Happiness is out there but the cheeky dickhead seemingly drives a newer model Mazda that breaks down heaps less and keeps getting away from us.

Black Girl in the Sundress

Anisa Nandaula

Black girl in the sundress.
Cry less.
With a drive to drive into car accidents called love less.
Hypocritic and helpless.
Convincing microphones that love poems mean something.
But my conscience is in an alleyway comforting sobbing hearts.
Saying words I don't mean to show feelings I don't have.
I prey.
      Then I pray.
I lie.
      Then I lay.

Black girl in the sundress.
Jobless.
Holding faith together with safety pins and calling it progress.
They say peace of mind is priceless.
But I just can't afford it.
Trying to buy a blue-collar tie
                  with a white college lie.
Living on the top floor of a tower made of bills.
Jumping out the window using this degree as a parachute.
Mama praying I fly.

Black girl in the sun dress.
Eating less.
Bones protruding from skin trying to confess
that I starve racing heartbeats and earthquakes from my body.
I am a house caught in a cyclone of panic attacks.

Choosing to live in the storm because destruction is a neighbour my
    body knows well.
Hunger is the bus route I take every day to university.
My body knows it well.

Black girl in the sun dress.
She is midnight wearing broken hearts, insecurity and hunger like
    stars.
Camouflaged in a smile carrying the sky around her hips.

Black girl hiding in the sun.

Three poems

Lotovale Junior Nanai

the stairway to heaven
the mind..
the body..
the culture..
the resistance..
the acupuncture..
now move or get hit..
the demons are liking you..
to offence the project to its company..
is results of conscience..
so salute the asteroid..
sorry bro don't get in my way..
or I will remove your course of passage..
that's just for starters..
amen

depression
the voice of the demon inside your noggin,
is the reminder of what pressure builds up by physicality,
and the mind twitches through paranoia,
and to be voice of consistency,
is the Trump card of your saviour,
so to be safe of qualifications,
one must abide by truth,
and all the quotes of disbelief,
is the underdog of promise

love
creativity of plus measures,
are it's coincidence of pasture,
but to resist temptation,
is to que up for Centrelink,
but those penny's of illustrious meaning,
has no concern for love,
for love of money,
is too entertain value of love

Paleochannel

Omar Musa

I'll let you in on the metaphor early.

Kintsugi: the Japanese art of repairing broken ceramics by filling the cracks with precious metals, to make an object more beautiful than before.

It seems impossible to accept the axiom when he says it with sober-eyed intensity; my sponsor (like another) loves to speak of alchemy and quote Carl Jung – 'the shadow is 90% gold'.

In Lahad Datu, on the east coast of Sabah, there are alluvial deposits, once-were rivers called 'paleochannels', where people look for gold. Wikipedia says that paleochannels are of geological importance because they help us understand the 'movement of faults'.

Twelve Steps down to the paleochannel now. Layer cake of shame and revelation, midden of shell and bone, shit and sucked ciggie, unpurged long-drop toilet. I probe like a needle in epidermis, a bin chicken looking for chips – in those rooms at the back of churches, where knees bounce and coffee is sipped from styrofoam. There are others with lithified livers, who hit rock bottom and called out to a god they didn't believe in.

I drank so hard that I shat blood and became a me I hated.

I drank so hard, I was seeking death; the drink became the only god I knew, the fool's golden euphoria. I did not need to die to know Hell.

I never wore gold growing up. Gold was promised in paradise, I was told, but in this life, it is a gaudy and unbecoming adornment. So when I pierced my ears with it and draped myself in chains and brand-name cloth, when I swallowed ribbons of amber, it felt like heresy. But in some Muslim societies, in the 'Golden Age of Islam', gold was used to heal eyes and heart, and in the cauterisation of wounds.

She – I called her my Rose Gold Lover. Maybe even in those words the unfair, fuckboi expectation that a woman should exact golden repair. We only deepened the cracks, it turned out, and made more. When she left, she gave me a Jung quote and a book on Japanese wabi sabi. I threw it in a box. Years later, I found it again. It spoke of beauty in impermanence, transience, and kintsugi. A glowing easter egg, hidden on a page, discarded.

90% of the world's gold is created by a kilonova, when two neutron stars collide and create a cataclysmic explosion that sends debris through space and time, shimmering particles that end up compacted into bright treasure, somewhere in the paleochannel beneath my feet.

I am on my knees now. There are other things here – skulls and vertebrae. Uranium, lignite. Useful but brutal, they burn. But I must dig on. I seek to pan precious things from shadow: with these hands of clay, this heart that slowly revolves on the potter's wheel.

Point Of No Return

Melanie Mununggurr

Their bathroom – an Ensuite
Shower, enough for just one person
On good days it grows
To fit two
Screen between flushed face
       And deep breaths
Takes form of a stained glass window
decorated in manic crayon soap scribblings
       of a writer
Memories and heartache, and hopes for the future
rain from the shower she dissolves tears under
       a mother
trying to rewrite her story into a happier one

She closes her eyes
only starless skies, opens them
Still only darkness
Even through the blur of salt drenched eyes
The exception
Crimson paint that runs,   from openings on her thighs
          s
            s
            s
            s

A permanent entry in her diary of pain
A reminder
where she scrawls   'you, are a bad mother'

Negative affirmations torment her
Poking and prodding her like bullies in the playground
Daring her demons to come out and play

While in the distance
Muffled lyrics of NF's 'let you down' are on repeat
Blasting on Dre's Beats
Every word rapid heart beats
And the Shower screams
          and thuds
A cover-up as she screams and thuds
Thumps walls and chest

Collapses

A drenched pile of flesh
Sobbing
Snorting water
Searching in panic
          for a breath

Listerine regurgitates minties nostalgia
Devoured by the packet, on school camps and road trips
Memories that will outlive her
When she drank the mouthwash
A chaser to twelve Panadol
Was it enough to take her breath away?
Or just enough to make giving CPR more pleasant
   For her rescuer
The freshness masking the bitter taste of lemons she'd
never have strength to transform into – lemonade
She wishes she could taste the water once more
but it no longer quenched her thirst to live
And with her desire to leave this world, her tastebuds too
departed early

Breath-taking tightness of his hands
clenching her fallopian tubes
like reins
Controlling the way her uterus moves, claim
sperm is superior to carrier
Father superior to her
Words, needles in her skin
Her own blade
Her weapon to release the pain
Hot water is running out, steam subsiding
Once warm heart
       Now freezing
And the squeezing in her belly
Rings out final remnants of belief
She's a good mum
Down
the metal drain

The stench of rusted iron
Infused with cherry blossoms
Her bodies white blood cells
Surrender to the toxins
Mutated by the trauma, she swallows
Her last breath
Seeking refuge in the corner
Where musty mould has begun to fester
And in this moment
Her despair outweighs
Her children's laughter

my body is a window

Scott-Patrick Mitchell

i.

which is to say: if you lift me up i will let in a thousand
fragrant blooms   spring air to hold you

but here's the thing about trauma: it builds bars around being
so used to my body pressed against glass, voices muffled
breath fogging up pane: i have become proficient in writing
the word HELP   backwards

ii.

in a TV show where people dress up as drag queens
contestants are asked to name their inner saboteur

ladies & gentlethem, please welcome to the stage
Sid   it is short for Insidious

iii.

Sid says *have you ever thought about a brief career in tying
knots*

Sid says *what would happen if we lay down & never got
up*

Sid says *if ya wanna go, let's*   *go*

Sid is not my friend

iv.

defenestration is the act of throwing a body through
a window, but how can i throw this voice outside myself

remember   trauma builds bars around being

v.

the writer Anna Borges has called
this chronic passive suicidal
ideation

i call it up at least five times a week, involuntarily
on the weekend we hang out, paint each other's nails:
as i order the pizza it plans an escape route
                              i so want to escape this

vi.

so i go to therapy, do the work, write lists about all of the reasons
i want to live   & on all of them, your name appears twice

i head home realising that i may be a car doing 40-something
down the freeway of life, tyres balding, odometer in need
of the occasional tap   but
my radio heart can still sing & when i wind the window down
my palm catches wind & surely this is reason enough to keep
                                     going

vii.

i get home, fill bucket with soap & water, take down all the bars
squidgy clean each sheet of pain, go inside, turn on all the lights
so i am bright & shiny because   my body is a window & now

now   you can see me

Septic tank universe

Misha the maniac

I live in a rectangle and it is the purity of the world in which I live. The sea surrounds the sun-silver walls which slithers radioactive junkie degenerates. Sklaaaaaatch, skraaaaaaaawww, shhhhhhhhhhlaaap of the tearing and pouring of blood, flesh and lime cascading from blades.

BUZZZZZZZZZZZZZZ

The sun-silver walls SHOOT five metres to the sun of the kingdom.

Government instruments penetrate with see-rays and battle with blood cameras that spray psychoactive substances to diffuse and disorient the opponent.

'Tut-tut' I mutter. 'A warthog-in-mud tactic.'

Someone shouts from criss-cross metallic megaphones.

Government vehicles stride the sky with beeps, blips and clicks permeating from slits in the high-beam lights. The council cleaners strip the Government Manufactured & Crafted 1905-vintage wallpaper that is pasted onto the firmament. Waste is compressed into structure-cubes cut in 2cm intervals.

The dettol lake sucks up the dirt-germs sourced from a constellation of abscesses held in various city hospitals. The three-amigo checkpoints filter the scum-particles held in the backseat of a vomit-car dropped into the dettol lake.

Behind, moving electric benches support statues which secrete white blood cells magnified-physical 2000 times. Autoclaves line the edges of the horizon. Steam puff furtive.

'Steam the air and strip it bare, boys.'

All drugs anti-cover the 5-metre perimeter of my bedroom. All anti-this and anti-that. Anti-histamines, anti-biotics, anti-septics and anti-psychotics. But I have no need for any of these, rolling as my brain does, no contaminants required nor sprayed mind/fur-altering microbes. (they fill the shelves). It's all anti-life. But purity and sterility wash the hands that forsake the filth. Eyes in an evil (they pierce the mirror) to which I stare in Kafka horror. My body is completely encased.

I am becoming a germ.

Reduced

D.L. Marcus

Diagnosis: blank, avoidant, clandestine.
Still eats lunch on time.
Fancies Sunday afternoons alone.
Locks journals into closure.
Sticks fingers into-the-back-of-the-eye-socket to check
if the image was there.
Finds shallow openings, in the flesh.
Written in single lines.
Or pockets, filled with fingers.
The hunger of a forgotten organ.
Caught between some webbing and a string.

Voice: hard, rubbery, formed.
The shuddering fatness of the neck.
Stubble that peeks into greeting.
An expression of knowing, stability.
He says the words are not your own we go around
in circles we go around this way
that doesn't lend itself to truth you can't repeat
yourself it doesn't lend itself to truth
and slammed the door.

Bed: bolted, plastic, stale.
Dig into the ankle with twisted thumb.
Unreceptive with a side of beans and vegemite.
Tubes found at short notice.
Please put it in, I need that, the hurt is alive.
Down the hall, stockings are improvised, but not quite, as rope.

Moved: to another closed room.
Head turned, open the door. They're distracted by the phone.
Go, now! Shelter beneath a stranger's stairs.
You were there: you carved yourself in orange stone.

Another: staircase. Does the hatred ever dissipate?
Stare at the sobbing bitch in the advertisement.
Her vacuity, smacked like concrete.
Forget how to take blood, let it spill like cherries' spit.
She came back home; but a boy was drowning nearby.
Did-you-know-this-call-is-keeping-us-from-helping-the-boy.
Stupid girl.

Stay: inside.
Inside the head, inside the tall wall.
Inside; inside the head, inside the head inside the tall wall.
Can you get a ball over the wall let's try it will you join me
if I run away I can't see myself in the mirror
anymore my face isn't the same can you help if I leave I have
before but I found my feet taking me back home dear *God*!

But god is not, god is not, find a staple because god is not.

Moment: blank, avoidant, crazed.
Chased around the corridors, drop that.
Grab the face, open the mouth.
Please god, but god is not.

Justopenyourmouthwhywon'tyouopenyourfuckingmouthwhyareyou
doingthiscan'tyouseewhatyou'redoingjustgetinthefucking
cardon'tspitthatoutorI'lltakeyoubackIswear
tofuckinggodIwilltakeyoubackcomeherecomehere*now*!

A rope that is cut in half, watch it fall back.
I should have been the drowning boy.

Intricately and Intimately Fractured

Anthony Mannix

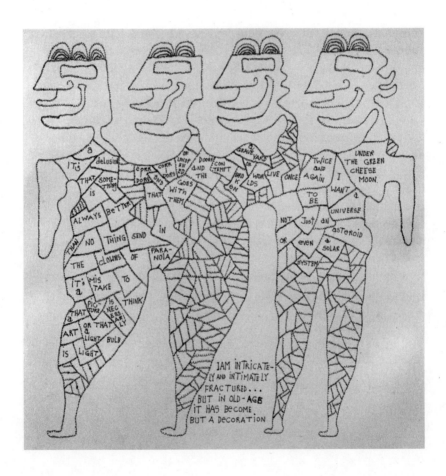

Metamorphoses and the Sunday of Life

Anthony Mannix

This is what in almost seven decades I have become. I am a perpetual anomaly, an oddity, like all of us.

Now I have four heads, four identities. It has been a slow change but it has happened. The body is fractured, intricately and intimately, but in one way it has become a brilliant decoration, and I do like decoration.

Words are part of the perception and decoration. I rely on them heavily. I was careful in the beginning but they have long since gotten out-of-hand, oozed out of the cracks in the box. I am not adventurous for the sake of being adventurous. I had to adjust but it is much easier that their weight is taken off my shoulders.

Now emptiness is everywhere but it sparkles; anyway it was always part of the landscape.

Inpatient (quite patient) XII

Gemma Mahadeo

You work for quantity [hours], activity [trying] to crack that object [nine-letter word puzzle] in object [newspaper] neatly copied onto object [ward whiteboard] for object [patients'] benefit.

- 1–9 words: good
- 6–20 words: very good
- 21–25: excellent
- 25+ words: inpatient, scrawls object [ward smart-arse]

I activity [smirk]; later activity [hate self] for activity [not being good enough] an inpatient.

If:
I: not present
at: morning community meeting
existence: accounted for?

I: present
at: here (hospital); not outside
existence: accounted for? please select:
    a. hospital or
    b. 'real'* life/world

Existence:
count: please select
a. outside or
b. inside (inpatient)?

admission: serious? please select severity:
a. no one who knows patient knows of admission
b. inpatient remembers entire admission
c. inpatient will be unlikely to recount admission in detail
*please note that because the inpatient is a patient at a private
psychiatric ward, all admissions are treated as voluntary*

(will my cat still remember me?
if i'm not feeding her everyday)

Inpatient:
- trying not to cry
- trying not to think about missing cat/animal companion/s whilst admitted
- can count semiquavers in complicated polyrhythms
- plays them slowly on melodica in room, or
- sneaks play of pianoforte in the adolescent ward recreation room

Inpatient is scared existence will count once discharged.
Inpatient is scared existence (they) will count once (they are) discharged.
I am scared existence will count once I am discharged.
I am scared my existence will count once I am discharged.
I am scared my existence will have to count once discharged.
I am scared my existence will have to count once I am discharged.
Inpatient is scared (their) existence will (have to) count once (they are) discharged.

* Healthy and rigorous debate about what constitutes 'real' life is encouraged and open to interpretation; please cite legitimate examples and include your sources.

Principal Diagnosis

Chris Lynch

A manic person rebels against the facticity of existence.
Moskalewicz & Schwartz (2020)

Start *in medias res* with the brilliant astonishment
of Persian red unrolling endlessly from beneath these

feet, the fractal displacement of the mundane,
                    the way the endless hallway improves

with a two-headed lamp, antler hatstand, and velvet green
armchair, the way the TARDIS transports you

from one floor of an apartment to another,
then returns you to an altered world, secretly parallel,

the way the immanent shadowy forest of a city park at 3am

is true, mute, moonlit, fertile, sledged, the way
the red brick in your hand could, if you so decide,

cave in your own skull. The decision tree, forking. Snakes.

End, instead, sitting cross-legged and serene

outside a petrol station, naked except for a blanket
discovered in the alley behind the vet.

Wait for enlightenment: inevitable
beneath the glowing yellow shell.

The blue man does not understand.
Does not, cannot, will not understand.

Enter the hospital like a king. Surgical gown. Antiseptic.
Psychoeducation about regen and self-referral

Odd presentation. FEels good, relaxed. (Imitially guarded).
Two way rational conversation able to recall
Normal flow rate and tone
Oriented to time, place and place
Arrived in a blanket
Remembers throwing keys in park
Denies ingesting mushrooms
Noted EMH handover differing from ED

Taken on lots of projects, gets lots of ideas but they , nil acute
Vague on interaction, disorganised, superficially pleasant and
polite, no agitation
Number given for wife goes through to HIS voicemail
Not able to recall why he took his clothes off but states it was
to save the world

Walking around cubicle talinf interst in all objects
Found knocking on doors
Ocasional loosening of associations. Kempt.
Lives alone, has multiple female friends
EMH were under the impression ED wanted to see him again.
Use sedation in the short term.

If with time these psychotic features do not attenuate
please feel free to re refer.

Grand flâneur

Rozanna Lilley

On the eve of his 20th birthday
I tell my son
there's a hole in his
favourite jellyfish T-shirt

The rest of it is still good
he objects   protecting his swarm
a peephole of pink skin
traversing sea & autumn sky

We clamber aboard
our waiting ark   washing up
at Grand Flâneur Beach
where Pathfinders bask

In Sunday formation
cheering pumped up jetskis
zigzagging an artificial lake
filling sandmine's scarred hollow

On shelter's strut
a black slash hastily
memorialises the last flood
muddy waters rising

A skein of trailing
tentacles weaving
the flotsam of our
shipwrecked intimacy

Cure

Kate Lilley

That first day on the street
you are standing outside your house
on the look-out

unexpected alliance
time given and taken
constant to inconstancy

the fear of existing
of not existing
receding

latch latched

Keep on Keep on

Nyaluak M Leth

Keep on   Keep on
You the king pawn in this board of duality

I mean   Actually
You the king prawn in the bucket of insanity

Keep on   Keep on
You got the keys to transform this reality

I mean   Actually
The secrets of the galaxies lie in your anatomy

To be reborn in your King form
You just gotta
Keep on   Keep on
For the you unborn

God ain't heard your sweet melodies in so long
Chile, won't you Keep on Keep on?
Go on, won't you sing for Him?

Little sister won't you   Keep on
Little brother won't you seek for Him
Oh Mama how you   Keep on Keep on Keep on

I speak form
Can't speak for em
We shift form and   Keep on – we
knock doors and   Reform – get
knocked down but We – Keep on Keep on Keep on

Bones

Luka Lesson

There are 206 bones in our bodies
and mine
are just like yours

but I'll be white ochre if I want to
I'll be bleached by sun and soaked by sand if I want to
I'll be eaten and reclaimed
decomposed and desired
if I want to

There are 22 bones in my feet
and I've named them after the poets who have walked before me

I will burn if I need to
be dust
if I choose to
desire smoke signals of yesterday
reminisce in my own future
I will be a figment of my own imagination if I choose to

I will be rubble
.drift wood
.dead weight
.dead set
.dead end
dead poet's society

There are 206 bones in my body
and each one will be fine bone china tea cup discussions
of what could have been
use my fibula to mark the chalk outline of what went wrong

reform my skeleton into a shape of something
you think you can come to terms with
like
how did he?
why did we?
why wasn't there?
when was it?
why didn't we?

There are 40 litres of water in our bodies
but most of us still can't find a fucking flow

I will build a dam if I want to
I'll build a river
an estuary
a lake

I will build a tear duct the width of your mother's face

I will not let her tell me we can't hear your voice anymore
I can't hear your voice any more than my own sometimes

My heart
beats
me up all day
and I know you know what that means

I know you miss me
but I wish you'd missed
And I'm not ready to shoot
the breeze with you

.not ready to fall with you
.not ready to flow
.not ready to go
.not ready to be that bold with you just yet
.not ready to decompose disintegrate or dissolve

I'm not ready to feed the dirt
just yet

as a poet
we're only ever respected once we're dead

                so I guess I'm not ready for fame just yet

I'd rather be anonymous – but breathing
Alive – in secret
a bad poet
but livid
average
but dealing with it

I'd rather be another number
than a statistic

        there is a difference

I'm not ready to fall just yet

There are one thousand miles of veins in our bodies
and I've given each vein a name
so when I'm gone
you still can't use my name in vain

And there are 36 breaths
in this poem
that I may have never taken
and they
are the best shit
that I ever wrote.

untitled

Jacinta Le Plastrier

(other)

           there are
      other
children,
               they are:
     not you (though
             your relative
       naked
would come to your
room)   yes,
        because
you survive–   just?
       you survived.
           childhood's lid,
   coffined

(limed)

                            you're
                               cornered, foetal.
                   there is no
                money, food no
the children bark.
         every thing, kept, rods
       away, lightninged. there is
       no greatness, no
petty.   in the limed light
                  of one dawn
            survive,   glow

Renovating Madness

Karen Knight

We can do a 60-minute makeover.
Spruce up the hollow-eyed
dormitories and bleached out
bathrooms, just like reality TV.

Let's start by removing the bars
on every window
putting back handles
on all the doors.

Expose the high-beam
hanging posts. Set up speakers
and pipe untroubled music
throughout the place.

Strip the wards
of canvas body holders.
Bulldoze the bed rails
and solitary restraints.

We'll brighten up the brickwork
the shadiest of corners.
Mend all the misery
within.

Core Sample

Krissy Kneen

I am learning about time
simultaneously
unlearning
everything that held me
fast to the earth.
Fast as a
lullaby,
spinning
safe as gravity
or the arms of a father
in that sweet brief moment when he burned
too bright
and collapsed into himself.

I am learning about time
from men
who look nothing like my father
who remind me of his absence.
Their guarded enthusiasm
when they say:
everything entirely exists
all at once
when they say:
ribbon
and
strip of film.

I think of a super-eight camera
celluloid sizzling
in the forge of memory,
in the spark of a miscalculated diagnosis,
in a whiff of migrainoid smoke.

Or perhaps time is here
by my side
or inside all at once
as my father is.
The years that are lost
are not lost
just cut up
and waiting
to be re-edited.

I am learning about time
and I can't keep all of it in my dumb head
and my brain takes on calcium
like a sea bed.
The tide seems to turn and turn again
ineluctably
every fold of new wave is
a layer of rockface.
Mind-rings like
core samples
the trunk of a tree
stretching back to
a laval earth.
The sound of it echoes
angry
through multiple connected universes
right down
to the moment
when my father left.

Since you asked

Paula Keogh

I want to learn the vernacular
of the world, feel the god of each thing
speaking through me

I want to say
oyster
eucalyptus
ice
and mean it

I want to close my lips around
the small bud of a noun and feel
the shape it will become

I want to release the words tangled
in my mind, say verbs that leap
from my throat, mend the broken
syntax lying in pieces on the floor

I want to say love without breaking,
say darkness and let it take me away,
let words catch fire
in the space between us

in the sandhills I want your voice
to cast a silver fish into the night
and say moonlight, say desire, more truly
than waves breaking

and in the morning on the veranda
I want to hear you speak
the unborn words floating
in your eyes, I want to unmute
my fears, cast spells, pray

but saying sanity won't heal me or even
put a roof over my pain, saying
bread won't bring you here
to share a meal with me

in the end, standing in a dark
corner of a world on fire, words
burnt to a crisp, what can be said?

the pilgrim has no place to go, and
this dreamer has
no mouth and
no voice

Tense

Lesh Karan

after Claire Gaskin's 'ahead'

The truth of where I am now is cicada-drowned: sullied surround sound. The truth of where I am now is rubber-band flicks in the cochlear: 24-hour snap-crackle-pop in the chamber. The truth of where I am now is white-water-raft fingers: monkeys in the mind steer my hull, then night falls and cracks sleep on my skull. The truth of where I am now is cortisol walking through a fog of fear in the atmosphere, seeking metamorphosis in a chrysalis of therapists. The truth of where I am now is *Lesh, do you want to be committed?* The truth of where I am now is box-breathing, deflated. The truth of where I am now is Zoloft and iPhone scaffolding the neurons, running from the self-portrait in every reflection. The truth of where I am now is bent-in-prayer for a past tense in the future. If only the truth would switch tunes: sing a lullaby, pacify the lizard pacing in my brain.

Results Day

Saanjana Kapoor

the ants have colonised   the white flesh of my half-eaten sandwich
I lean closer   water droplets from my hair leaving puddles   then
    a lake in their path
this is the golden age   but it's been Monday for weeks
my best friend stumbles inside   and I wonder if she would cherry-
    pick me now
we were each other's reflections   in the class of '17
myopic dreams tucked in our back pockets   heads crammed with
    fears
we cycled for hours under tie-dyed skies   to ogle at glass houses
    lining the beach
wished upon broken shells   ran before the shore returned them
braids swinging   tupperware thumping against our hips
    at every step
we'd carpool to school   to bow our heads over textbooks
    carpool home
to pirouette our fingers over keyboards
    until the morning's first light
this was the game we'd die to win   our hours like tokens
a handful stolen from a classmate's party
a couple from the unfinished movie
a single plucked from each skipped meal   until a marionette sits at
    a littered desk
its ears   a ballot box of their worst words
its eyes   a fishnet for my mistakes
its lips   a set of taut ropes   whose colonised wail
    silences my mother's
did I just spend thirteen years sharpening my silver tongue   only
    to curl it
into a bouquet of corporate cliches

the last day is a terminal   where not all the exits are visible   I sit
        in my school blazer
that I never grew into   it still feels cut for someone else
        as I wait at the airport bar   for results day
I never wanted anything   except a father's smile   but
this is the most ruthless magic trick I have ever seen
my life's work disappearing in front of me

Triptych: Post Traumatic Relationship Syndrome

Gabrielle Journey Jones

1. P.T.R.S.

Pretend you're okay
Tell no-one the truth
Relinquish identity
Stay small and silent.

Plan your escape
Try a few hundred times
Resist in secret ways
Scared and compliant.

People will help
This pain will pass
Re-enter the world
Solid steps of resilience.

Prepare your allies
Talk about defence
Reorganise your energy
Stage your insurgence.

Prioritise your safety
Trust your intuition
Realise your worth
Survive domestic violence.

2. Gaslit

They fashion
Makeshift weapons
From your unsuspecting words
Whatever you dare to say
Is used to beat you down
As if you attacked yourself.

Silence is what saves you.

They think
No-one will believe you
They ensure you're isolated
Remove your safest places
Favourite people first
You imagine you're alone
Then they attempt their worst.

They want
Their actions to hurt
Emotional violators
Coercive control abuse
Is not a new method
to redefine your truth.

Compliance is what hides you.

3. Edges

Edge of truth
Edge of tears
Edge of comfort
Edge of queer.

Two-edged sword
Two-way street
Two-toned souls
Two-fold relief.

Folded arms
Folded hearts
Folded stories
Folded cards.

Cards held close
Cards ignored
Cards unplayed
Cards overthought.

Overexposed
Overcome patterns
Overtly content
Overdue joy.

The Madwoman in this Poem

Sandy Jeffs

After Bronwen Wallace

For Gudrun
Yet how stupendous a psychosis
in which God is heard...
Gudrun Hinze

The madwoman in this poem
lives on the twenty-second floor
of a block of flats
her husband and children gone
each day she waits for a letter
that never comes
her wrists carry a flurry of scars
her arms are dotted with cigarette burns
every day she contemplates jumping.

The madwoman in this poem
walks the streets
reciting Shakespeare and Milton
she shelters in bus stops and doorways
scrounges through rubbish bins
drinks from discarded beer bottles
begs for money to buy cigarettes
and a moment's respite.

The madwoman in this poem
slumps into a ramshackle chair
hiding herself
her large torpid body founders
her heavy breasts gush
drug-induced lactation

her body grows
with each anti-crazy pill
she reluctantly swallows.

The madwoman in this poem
transfixes in front of the TV
absorbing its many messages
Ally McBeal is her daughter
Eddie McGuire can read her mind
Ridge and Brooke are talking to her
are going to come in a helicopter
take her to Venice to meet Brad Pitt.

The madwoman in this poem
lives in a holy grotto
awaiting the Pilgrims
she carries the burden of Eve
smells God in the toilet
sees the Virgin above the lintel
has given birth to the New Messiah
carries the secret of the Holy Grail in her heart
was raped by the Devil
sees maggots wriggling in her stigmata.

The madwoman in this poem
is sure Beethoven stole the
nine symphonies from her
cannot walk on the cracks of the pavement
can feel spiders eating her brain
fears her head is about to explode
is going to the firing squad next morning
is a character in a Bruegel painting
is an oracle of the dead.

The madwoman in this poem
is everywoman
is any woman
is a mother, daughter,
sister, lover, friend—
the madwoman in this poem —
is me.

People Die in Seclusion Rooms

Anna Jacobson

Woman lies face to feet
under a white sheet on a bare
concrete floor in a bare
concrete room.

Walls say: *Another one.*

Woman is dead, the staff
did not watch. No one wants to
watch a woman who cannot watch
for herself.

Walls say: *We are the watchwomen.*

She fell many times and hit
her head on a bare concrete floor
in a bare concrete room. That woman
could have been me.

What do you want, padded walls? says Nurse.

Walls say: *We want all soft edges and no room.*

Doc looks me in the eyes.
*You were placed in seclusion
many times, more than most.
Do you remember this?*

No, I don't remember.

I was not there in my self while my body
lay on the bare mattress and screamed
for my return.

Nurses made brief records – un-watching
the woman who cannot watch for herself.

Hospital file tells me I smuggled
in a pen. Security assisted. The pen
was removed. I wrote on the floor with cold
cups of tea. My words were not noted –
no one wants to listen to the woman
who cannot hear herself.

They removed the bedframe in case
I hit my head. But what of the bare concrete
floor in a bare concrete room filled
with ghosts of those from before?

I don't remember the seclusion room.
Though a part of my self still haunts
its walls, floor, page.

Brittle

KJ

i

Slow. Slowly—my sense of self slipping through the seams that sew
us together.
Us. Me. Wife. Mother. A sewn-on patch of horizontal-striped
solidarity.
Disintegrating—friable, a human-shaped plastic weathering in the
sun and flaking away.

ii

Was it when I was crawling up the back of the chair?—Watch out.
Maybe I was breathing and not breathing and my teeth were
breathing.
Staring as my veins enlarged—look at the blood on the mirror.

iii

Escorted to my room—My packed-the-day-before bag holds my hand
Inside the remnants of my sanity.

iv

The doctor of discomfort. I am transparent and I cannot deflect.
Reflect.
Elbows to knees to x-ray my brain with his eyes.
In/Two/Months/Time/You/Will/Have/Either/Killed/Yourself/Or/
You/Will/Be/Back/Here
Do I have the receipt for that 'Choose Your Own Adventure'?

v

One-woman #cancelculture—my career of twenty-six years. Gone.
When I look in the mirror. Where's the mirror?
I share and crawl and shake uncontrollably. There are consequences.

Loss of identity—No other truth.
Invisible in my mirror. She. My wife. Can she be my mirror?

vi
My mental and physical at war. Raze Race.
There is no yin and yang. There is just y.
Wrenching, searing, silent detonating sobbing—drain the last of that milkshake
The gift of a stomach-ache from a thousand sit-ups.

vii
A glance. Meagre scraps of myself
Paltry dust bunnies and bereaved lint in shadowy corners where
I had sometimes looked—never looked—-always looked.
Perhaps now to trust the sunlit sequins and glitter.

viii
Collect. Stoop and pinch.
There is room in a pocket of my heart.
Stickers and showtime lights around the edge of my mirror.

Comic Sans

Holly Isemonger and Chris Fleming

This is your form
If you make a mistake, don't
cover it up

So, This is a form again.

Straighten your back.

Focus and start.

Don't be sneaky.
Use only blue or black pen.

I have stencils backdating my failures
Capital letters itemise time, tide, trauma
In other words, do you have
a green, purple or light blue pencil?

A momentous choice.

Put the pen in the bag, remove the bag, put it on,
light it up and charcoal the beast you arrived on.
Find and follow the dot.

It's been more than 10 years now
Don't let anyone see that
your pen is older and you are not

Sure enough, go out and buy a cheapskate pen
choosing the right item is an important choice,
a moustache, a suit, a collar?

In the loud voice
of men—'Can I have a pen? Is this true?'

Then go back and fill this out:
What kind of handwriting is this?
Looks like writing for the beach.

First impressions matter
You are talking
Separate and use handwriting.

I admit I blew it up.

Why do I still use that font?
If you have a wound salt water will aid the healing;
if you have a beach the tide will erase
the whole thing.

I wish you good luck.
But Jesus, what's on the page?

A victim who feels like a villain

Martin Ingle

I was preparing to get onstage at the Sydney Opera House and I couldn't stop thinking about the excruciatingly real possibility that I might like the taste of human flesh.

Needless to say I had never tasted it before. But that didn't matter. How did I *know* I didn't like it? My mind scanned back over every memory throughout my whole life of any articles I'd read or any stories I'd heard about cannibals, trying to retrospectively analyse my reactions to them. Was this something I had always secretly wanted? Outrageous, obviously…*but isn't it possible, Martin? Why not?* Oh God. Had I been subconsciously hiding this horrendous cannibalistic desire inside that I was only now aware of because I had stumbled across the question? Is this who I really am?

Hold on. Why is this thought even occurring to me?! Why can't I find a resolution to it? And now when I take a bite into a delicious piece of meat why can't I stop thinking about it being human? A thought so horrible I want to spit it out right away! But for some reason it won't go away when I tell it to.

This is just one example of a terrifying phenomenon, a sort of thought virus that unbeknownst to me had incubated in my brain a couple of months before this and had quickly grown to infect my entire life. In the winter after I turned twenty-three, I had begun to truly lose control of my thoughts. It started sneakily, a parasite in the shape of a question mark that when fed very quickly grew and took over my mind completely. I didn't know it at the beginning, but these thoughts were the loose threads that, timidly tugged, would soon unravel me.

If I could be afraid of it, then this thought monster could accuse me of it. Cannibal, sure. But that's easy stuff. How about murderer? Psychopath? Abuser? Liar? The most disturbing for me are the sexual ones – fears that I might want to harm people pale in comparison to fears I might get unconscious sexual pleasure from it; that I'm secretly, fundamentally, incurably broken; so secretly I don't even know it. Paedophila? Beastiality? Incest? Rape? Oh yeah, my terrified brain has thrown it all at me, scrolling rapidly through every horrible possibility like the slots of a pokie machine, desperately searching for evidence that I'm dangerous so I can protect the world from myself, the content of the thoughts limited not by the strength of my stomach but by the impish creativity of my fearful mind. Very quickly I grew this remarkable and basically uncontrollable superpower to think the extreme and catastrophic worst of myself. It's like being an anti-Kanye. Kanye East.

Of course, because I hated this whole damn situation so much, I had cast it out, to prove it wrong, to prevent any of these uncontrollable thoughts somehow becoming uncontrollable actions. After a few relentless years of these ever-growing extreme measures, though, I could hardly function. I lost work. I lost relationships. At my worst, I could hardly eat. Pants started falling off me. I didn't masturbate for six years, and I went a year and a half as a neuter with no sexual release at all. My hands were cracked and bursting at the seams. To avoid the toilet I would pee hands-free into the bathtub. No shit. (Oh yeah, I avoided shitting too.)

When it started, I thought these things were the only way to remain a somewhat intact human being and avoid sure catastrophe – like pouring cold water on a scalding thought. But once it got a hold of me, this thought monster just about took over. It twisted the beautiful into the obscene. It hijacked the things in my life that I most valued and distorted them in the worst ways imaginable.

Without much warning, the thoughts in my mind went rogue. They turned against me and mutinied. The result is nothing short of constant daily torture. Before this my biggest fears used to be an imagined or vague future. Now they are in everything I think and everywhere I look: behind the next page in a book; the next click of a mouse; a word, a number, a memory, a thought, a doubt; behind my eyelids in the morning before I jerk myself awake. They are with me at every moment of every day, not just possible but immediate, not just future but present. At best it's a thorn you can't get out; a mosquito in the back of your brain that you can't kill. My thoughts are essentially out of my control, the brake lines cut and I'm swerving. It's basically the cruellest prison for your mind you can imagine, and the best part is it's made specifically for you – because it's made by your own brain.

I didn't know it when this all started, but this horrific thing has a name.

Obsessive Compulsive Disorder.

You've heard of OCD right? That's the one where your house is spotless, right? The one where you have to line your pens up perfectly, right? The one where you wear surgical gloves all the time or are afraid of getting sick or only eat the purple M&Ms or something, right?

Well, no. I don't do any of those things. Your traditional image of somebody with OCD – hunched over a sink scrubbing their hands – crudely describes only some OCD sufferers, and even then doesn't begin to tell the real story.

My psychologist can explain it better:

'OCD means having awful, scary, unwanted thoughts, images or urges that barge into your mind, and that the more you try to get rid of them, the more they come. Despite your best attempt to reduce, manage or prevent these scary thoughts or images, they take up residence in your mind, wreaking emotional havoc.'

I found Dr Clare Rosoman after timidly disclosing my unwanted thoughts to two separate therapists who were unable to tell me what was wrong with me. Luckily for me, she knew about true OCD and confirmed what until then only Google had told me. By that point, my mind had descended to the darkest places imaginable, on one hand terrified I was an evil pervert and on the other hand screaming that I wasn't – *there was no proof! Was there?* And all this was happening behind my eyes.

If you're confused, I don't blame you. If you're disturbed, join the club. This description of OCD runs contrary to almost everything we think we know about it, and instead draws an unrecognisable but somehow eerily familiar picture of what is perhaps the world's most misunderstood mental illness.

As I learned over the following years, the 'obsession' part of OCD can actually latch on to any subject at all. Sure, fear of germs might be one, but there are literally countless others. These are often extreme and, for lack of a better word, 'taboo' topics (sex, violence, crime, immorality), but can also range to the abstract and metaphysical (*Am I real? What even is reality?*).

English writer Rose Cartwright was one of the first people I heard publicly talk about this specific kind of OCD. Her watershed article in *The Guardian* in 2013 telling her story curiously dropped a month or two after my own OCD began, all the way across the other side of the world. (Even more curiously, it was also this exact same year that the American Psychiatric Association reclassified OCD as its own unique illness, rather than having it fall under the general umbrella of anxiety disorders. Turns out 2013 was a lucky number for obsessives like me.)

In her article and the book that followed, Rose Cartwright talks about the darkness of living undiagnosed with this kind of OCD (nicknamed 'Pure O') as feeling like you have a body buried in your backyard and nobody knows except you. You are expected to go on living a life normally – reading the daily paper, going to work, taking a lunch break, calling your mother – you are doing all these really mundane or perhaps even enjoyable things, all while this body is buried in your backyard.

You feel like a pretender. Like maybe you are that guy who moves to a small town and everybody thinks is really nice until they discover he was a serial killer on the run and was skinning cats in his bathtub while singing Wagner or something. You fear *that is you*. And you despise it. But you can't stop thinking it.

I found myself living two lives at once: the one inside and the one outside my own head. At its worst it could feel like I was in a dream, witnessing my actions and conversations as if I was an invisible first-person audience member to my own life. In conversations I felt like I was just on autopilot. I could have entire interactions with people and have my mind constantly whirring manically over an unrelated thought while at the same time having a completely different and normal conversation in the real world.

I carried this weight with me all the time, a thick wet blanket behind my eyes, smothering me. Living in that grotto of doubt is suffocating. The air is thicker there. Your thoughts are custard. And you're not swimming, you're drowning.

My personality felt like a shallow performance, a memory of how I once was that I was reconstructing for the world's benefit. All while, on the inside, I was a total mess. No matter how I tried, there was no forgetting or turning off these thoughts, and I sure as hell didn't want to let them show on the outside.

The thoughts presented themselves as problems to be solved, and were so important that I felt obligated to try to resolve them so I could move on. It's just that the moving on never happened. The resolution was never really there. The solution was never concrete and sure, even when logically I knew that it must be, somehow. The evidence was all there in front of me, but it was like having cataracts on your brain. You can see what must be the truth, but it's murky as hell and you certainly wouldn't operate heavy machinery.

So no – obsessive compulsive disorder really is nothing like you think. To say that OCD is about cleaning is like saying the flu is about blowing your nose. No, this is really about thoughts: intrusive thoughts that we all have, but that the OCD brain can't turn off.

Lee Baer subtitles his iconic (my OCD tells me 'seminal' is too sexual) book *The Imp of the Mind* as *Exploring the Silent Epidemic of Obsessive Bad Thoughts*. The Silent Epidemic.

We know that virtually everyone has intrusive thoughts – and they are universal in content. Sex, violence, blasphemy, they are the same across the board in healthy and unhealthy people alike. Obsessive compulsive disorder is the next step: how you react to those thoughts.

It's thought one in fifty people has OCD, with other claims varying to as high as 5 per cent of the population. It's hard to say exactly how many people have it, as the content of intrusive thoughts often fills people with intense shame, so it's the last thing you want to talk about. Instead you suffer in obsessive silence, just like I did, but for others it can be for literally decades: it takes an average of *seventeen years* before someone with OCD finds the right treatment. In retrospect, I got off easy.

And yet OCD is still seen as a fringe illness, basically only affecting quirky but loveable weirdo characters in movies and people on reality TV hoarding shows. The kind of thing for water cooler talk, like that documentary you saw last night about the guy whose fingernails are six feet long or the woman who was in a coma from eating an expired croissant and can now speak French and recognise photos of herself from the 1800s.

This incorrect perception of what OCD is has real, tangible effects on these silent sufferers who don't even realise they're sufferers. When my thought spirals began, nobody would have been able to tell anything was wrong at all from the outside. I know I didn't. I wasn't cleaning compulsively or turning a light switch off and on again. But I didn't need to be – I was seriously ill with something the World Health Organization once famously listed in the top ten most disabling illnesses in the world. I just didn't know it.

The journey to finding out you have OCD is long and exhausting, but this is only the start. Talking about it is the next big step, or rather a big heavy bastard of a door that you timidly open crack by crack. Talking about my intrusive thoughts with my psychologists was one push of that door. What you're reading right now is another. Don't be fooled by how solid this seems in black and white. I remain sick and scared, and on the delicate edge of life-destroying risk.

I've only recently started to talk about my intrusive thoughts so graphically (not to mention publicly), and I'm terrified of the effect it could have on my life. Make no mistake, the potential consequences are catastrophic. When any future first date googles my name, what on Earth will they think? Will my current employers at my day job – both Christians – find a reason to stop giving me shifts, secretly thinking I'm a pervert who shouldn't interact with their customers? How can I ever show my face at a family gathering again with them knowing these things that have been in my head for almost a decade? Who will ever let me in front of their children again? Their pets? How can I ever allow *myself* these things?

I've had to let go of a lot of these dreams. I've had to grieve this imaginary life path that I now only walk adjacent to. Maybe in another world I could have lived it. Maybe one day I still will, who knows? For now, I'm a watchful, day-dreaming ghost, haunting a happier version of a man who doesn't even exist.

At this point you might find yourself asking what is to me a familiar question: how do you know the difference? How can you know somebody who has obsessive thoughts about sex crimes is not a potential sex offender, or that the person with intrusive violent thoughts won't one day snap and murder someone? Funnily enough, this question is most often asked not by outsiders like you, but by OCD people themselves desperate to find reassurance from the thoughts that they hate.

Dr Scott Blair-West is a psychiatrist who runs the inpatient treatment program for OCD sufferers at The Melbourne Clinic. To this question, he has the obvious clinical answer that he's seen play out time and time again:

'I'm always confident that OCD people are not dangerous because it's always clear that the intrusive thoughts/images are always completely the opposite of what the person wants to do AND they are really upset about even having the intrusions. We call the intrusions/obsessions ego-dystonic, i.e. against the ego.'

It's no wonder to me why people with OCD keep their thoughts to themselves. I have, until now. It's no wonder why people with OCD are ten times more likely to attempt suicide than the general population. They hate their unwanted thoughts more than anyone. They are more likely to believe they are evil than anyone.

I wonder how many die by suicide before even discovering they have OCD; where their intrusive thoughts have bombarded them in secret for so many years that they are convinced they are evil, when they are actually just ill. My heart aches for those people: victims of their own brain, forced to feel like villains. Carrying all the guilt, having committed none of the crimes.

Dr Rosoman goes even further:

'I would have to say that of all the people I have the privilege of working closely with in my practice, people with OCD are the most kind, sensitive and intuitive. They tend to be highly intelligent and to be extremely creative thinkers', she says. 'They are beautiful people, tortured by their worst fears.'

So: how to escape from this living hell of your own brain's creation?

In a small ward on the first floor of The Melbourne Clinic you'll find around a dozen or so obsessive compulsive disorderlies tackling treatment for many different kinds of OCD. It remains the only inpatient treatment program for OCD in Australia, and is run by Dr Blair-West, who is straightforward and clinical and to me the kind of guy you see when you look up 'psychiatrist' in the dictionary. When it comes to OCD, he's seen it all. He agrees to meet with me and show me around the program.

Treatment for OCD is both deceptively simple and unimaginably torturous. Exposure with Response Prevention (ERP) is the gold standard, and involves being guided by a trained therapist through 'exposures' to whatever your fear/obsession is. Naturally, your anxiety will skyrocket, particularly if it's a highly feared obsession, but that's where the 'response prevention' comes in: you must *not do the compulsion* and instead wait for your anxiety to naturally decline. Over time – anywhere from minutes to months – your brain habituates, and the thought eventually causes no anxiety at all.

It's the equivalent of asking an arachnophobe to hold a tarantula on their face until it doesn't bother them anymore.

ERP is the exact kind of treatment that Dr Blair-West and his team at The Melbourne Clinic guide the OCD group through as part of their three-week inpatient course. This morning they are venturing out of the clinic to the local park for a sort of exposure field trip. They each have their own individual exposures to do while we're there: anything from walking past a stranger to patting a dog or touching a gate. Tame for you maybe, but for them, excruciating.

Their treatment is tailored to each of them, but it's the same fundamental principle no matter what their obsession is. Sex, violence, health, religion – it doesn't matter here. OCD treatment teaches that there is essentially no difference between 'mild' topics like contamination and more disturbing subjects like fear of paedophilia. The *content* of your intrusive thoughts is meaningless – the illness is exactly the same across the board, for all these people. This explains how my OCD brain has been able to so easily jump from obsession to obsession over the years. *Am I a cannibal...Am I a sexual pervert...Did I just hit someone with my car...Do I really love my girlfriend or am I just pretending...*All these vastly different topics don't matter. The things I'm obsessing about aren't real; the illness fuelling all of them is.

This, however, is a hard pill to swallow. Lord, give me *anything* except this. Give me *any* thoughts except these. I'll take anything else. Do not make this my burden. I've yelled at a God many times over the years, keeled over and caked in sweat, stuck in an inescapable thought spiral. I don't pray; I don't believe; but I still beg Him, call Him, curse Him, perhaps out of habit if nothing else. He doesn't come. I am still sick.

I'm joining the inpatients in their exposure trip to the park today not as a sufferer but a writer – not to be treated, but to observe. But even simply being here with them is my own exposure. I grit my teeth as I chat with their guiding psychologist, all while silently feeling that familiar thumbscrew tightening in the back of my mind; we are standing next to an empty playground and I hope people don't suspect we are sex offenders waiting for prey. I'm careful not to touch anything either. Any other day I would do anything to avoid the playground completely – cross the road, even take absurd side streets in a circle to avoid walking anywhere near it – but today I am empowered to sit with my pain just like the rest of the disorderlies around the park who are similarly choosing to suffer through their own.

ERP has a success rate of around 70 per cent in most people and, in conjunction with medication, can help people short-circuit the loop of fear and reaction that OCD traps you in. How sad that the mental illness I was once terrified of telling anyone about is also the one that is most treatable.

Even the best treatment is unlikely to remove intrusive thoughts entirely, though. It has been almost eight years for me and while I've been through many different therapies and am still on medication, it hasn't totally gone away. Part of living with OCD involves accepting the grief of those lost years.

OCD forces you to live face to face with your worst imaginings. Our outrage at these thoughts is extreme – more extreme than anyone's – and our reaction to them disproportionate and pathological. It doesn't mean we care more, it just means we lack the process in our brain that enables us to care less. Your process. The normal process. Because no matter how much your average person cares, at some point you *have* to switch off, you *have* to let go. Otherwise you would never drive a car again.

If you don't have OCD, these topics probably still disturb you to even think about, and rightly so. But we disorderlies – at least those of us who have been through the appropriate therapy – have a secret about this: no matter how dark, how dangerous, how hurtful, how traumatic these thoughts are, they remain, always, just thoughts. Nothing more. Ideas. They can't harm us. Therapy for OCD teaches you exactly this: to accept the uncertainty, the chaos, the inexplicable nature of our brains. We with OCD know that we can't cushion ourselves against a sharp world. And for those of us who get obsessed with every horrible possibility, we shouldn't. It only makes us sicker.

But it can change. It did for me, almost immeasurably. It does get better. If you keep going for long enough, hope starts to peek its timid head out from behind despair.

Because even through countless setbacks, even through the daily slog of uncontrollable waking nightmares, and through nights of drunk-like mental headcolds, I eventually always got out the other side. I learned that no matter how dark it gets, if I just wait for long enough there is always a way out. Especially if I can't see how at the time. Somehow. Somehow. Somehow you find a way.

The future is a horizon curved beyond your sight.

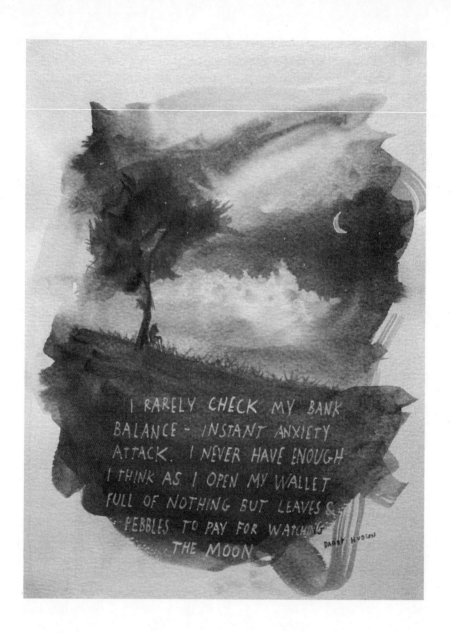

I RARELY CHECK MY BANK
BALANCE - INSTANT ANXIETY
ATTACK. I NEVER HAVE ENOUGH
I THINK AS I OPEN MY WALLET
FULL OF NOTHING BUT LEAVES &
PEBBLES TO PAY FOR WATCHING
THE MOON

DARBY HUDSON

100 Points of ID to Prove I Don't Exist

Darby Hudson

- Some dream I wrote on a scrap of paper (10 points)
- Syncing my watch to the distant sound of a barking dog (18 points)
- Letting all my bills get eaten by snails (23 points)
- Shazaming the wind in the trees (4 points)
- Recognising that walking a dog on a long leash is really just flying a ground kite (2 points)
- The bottomless void of a no text response silently crushing a planet (73 points)
- Drinking water collected only by night (26 points)
- Patting a stray cat and keeping a bit of its fur that accidentally stuck to my hand (14 points)
- Eating a peanut butter sandwich in the shower and not telling anyone (25 points)
- Realising that writing poetry is really just writing one really long suicide note your whole life before dying of old age (113 points)
- Calling my name into a crowd and seeing if anyone responds (150 points)
- Losing my name, calling for it, and it never returning (300 points)
- I enter a room, the room enters me, I vanish (438 points)
- Walking backwards into the future – to not leave a trail – so you can never find me (500 points)

three approaches to mem*ry

Ruby Hillsmith

1.

i feel the hot/shock of the silver hook

and nurse it for a little while

before i even check—(*which bastard's*

reeling in the fishing line?)

and that's just the curse of mem*ry:

sometimes it turns the gut
                    before the throat
                            before the eye

(*that one delinquent pupil always seems to trail behind*)

and now i want to give up history,

the pit of broken glass

i drag my fingers through
                      (and then revise, each

tiny prick a patient under mem*ry's super/vision)

to get a job on *neighbours*: chief amnesiac,

a girl and her huge plot hole.

2.

i cross the border without breaking

mem*ry's autocratic state.

the body keeps the score, and

melbourne's nice, it's just another place

to drag the chariot,
                            to blather on and on before

old visions come in threes—*still*—

there is the mosquito bite i pick until it bleeds,

currents gripping me
                            (((parentheses))),

mangroves twisting like a mess of snakes towards the sun.

i hire a dodgy contractor to start the demolition—

he says grief is an expan$ive lot to be developed

into westconnex and reams of wet cement

(*that you can barely press your palms against*
                            without a fine)

3.

mem*ry arrives, again———(((*as if it bears repeating*)))

you:
    impudent in a cowboy hat,

worn tracksuit

dyed a fetching shade of pink—
                                granted—a

mem*ry has to change a bit each time it's resurrected,

so you've burned through all your outfits pretty quick—

and all at once I beg the past

to skim my chest

without incision,

indifferent as a bar of motel soap—

(((but))) suddenly the faucet turns

(((and))) someone's calling down the hall

(((like))) *slash the ribbons, hurry on*

short of a witness———mem*ry's gone———

for finn

Ruby Hillsmith

///and
one day i'll be happy///and
we'll fucking live it up,
one day I'll float through your brick house
like nothing///no-one ever cracked me///
there are strange graces
in this trouble
but i've had to eke them out,
tried on the patience of a saint
((ha)
spending all my time
in///habit(s))
///and finn
of course—
right now the dream feels far///
but today
there is the poem
there is the dancing veil of rain
there is my friend across the border
there is my friend
///there is
///there is

from the book of puns and other altered sentences

Tim Heffernan

(sutherland hospital, april 2020)

i
the blue chair is algorithmic and we who are not apostrophes
cannot spoil the things we do with the furniture
we love useless things, so if you are digging with a spoon
in the garden of the hdu and you are a poet and mad
remember it is a spoon and not a pen

ii
in the morning, in the muralled hospital courtyard
a star, the mourning star points down
in the afternoon, the sun contrives with the sail cloth
to create a specific volcano

iii
it is twenty minutes since you took your meds
zyprexa, the communion wafer
the blasphemous one
instead of taking it on the tongue
you take it under the roof of your mouth
sedative tongue kisses numbing us

iv
leaving the tomb on the third day you try
to stop them thinking you are end dead
but if you don't want to say anything
just go and know you'll come back

out the front of the caravan park
where no one can hear us
just you and me pressing against time

v
there are always devils on the ward
they spit bullets into the mouths
of the innocents and drag us down
with their growling, clawing, gnawing syllables.
there are always angels on the ward
they speak flowers at medication time
watering our tomorrows. they lift us up
with their songs, their wings, and their beautiful caresses

vi
it is the coming down time
coming down from the vision place
the reminder of concrete landings and the smashing of intellect
it is the fool tripping over his outrageous shoes
again, again & again

vii
it is like history playing backwards
what has been done is
playing live – music improvised
the future catches up with the past
and in time you are moving
back and forward to your present

viii
to get out of here we all need to walk to schedule
meals arrive on dalek-trays vertically mirroring
the ward where the rooms are stacked laterally
unlike their inhabitants. it's still all about screen-time
nurses stare out of the fishbowl while we swim round and round

ix
on each of our leave breaks
a newly born baby emerges from the
hospital entrance/exit into this Covid-19 world
evidence that this day belongs to them
as we sit on the grass seeking distance
from each other

Frequency

Jenny Hedley

excavate / integrate
dense memories[1]
warped record
broadcast radio
shame on repeat[2]

    ur device is not connected
    make sure 'Jenny' is turned on
    & in range
    now discoverable as 'Jenny'

b4 violence : laughter
attacks   / unbearable
gumballs / bubble
baths   / curious
razors / cuddle
toys / edelweiss

'Jenny' v2.0 =
blind retinal degeneration
numb pelvis hungry
hollow wilful swallow

    not connected
    connection unsuccessful
    connected
    ur connection is unstable

oral fixation
/ dehydration /
failure 2 articulate
/ bellyache[3] /

Thinking is drilling

Justin Heazlewood

I'm drilling through the walls
of silence and confusion
looking for clues
looking for answers
looking for Mum.

I have a lot of
work to do.

So I sit and I stare
and I think so hard
I can cut through the moon
because I'm the sun.

Thinking is drilling.

I'm drilling up and out of the rubble.
Thinking is making air for myself.
A space to survive.

I can think into space
into outer space
into inner space.
I can drill inside
deep down and hide.
I can drill around in circles
so fast that everything's a blur
and I have rings like Saturn.

A drill is a weapon
with a pointy tip.
I leave it running
to rip the black pillows
when they come to smother me.

Thinking is drilling.

My mind is always moving.
There's work to be done
a maze to be dug
a tunnel of fun
somewhere deep
to bury my time capsule.

Retreat

Amani Haydar

1.

Trauma; a psychological wound. In Arabic, *sadma*; a sudden shock, impact, jolt. The thing you can't unsee. Triggers take biological form in the brain. Grooves in a snowy slope, skis digging deeper and deeper. Howling canyon between hemispheres. Slippery brain, spongy brain, molten brain. Left brain disconnected from right. Brain disconnected from body. Brain disconnected from breath.

I decided to attend a trauma recovery retreat for survivors of domestic violence because a sadness I thought I could outrun caught up and seeped in. I had just finished writing and editing my book and we were in the midst of the pandemic. Realisations I'd made while writing had unearthed new griefs or, perhaps, new ways of looking at the same grief. I found myself listening to My Chemical Romance like it was 2007 and re-watching episodes of *Glee* while eating 2-minute mi goreng.

2.

Fifteen women attended the retreat, each of us differently harmed by a man, or two, or several. We sat in a circle on the floor of the ashram. In the middle was a quilt decorated with crystals, cards and candles. The facilitator introduced herself and instructed us to set our intentions by lighting a candle and focusing on one word that represented our hopes for the weekend. One by one, around the circle, women introduced themselves and stated their intentions: 'Joy', 'Safety', 'Confidence'.

'Calm,' I said firmly as I lit my candle. 'My intention this weekend is to find calm because I have not felt calm in a long time.' As the remaining women took their turns, I wondered about the crystals arranged at the centre of the quilt, sceptical about their alleged healing properties. It did strike me, however, that these objects had formed in volcanoes, hidden in rock, buried deep in the Earth's ancient crust. There was no natural or biological reason that they should be beautiful, yet they twinkled as though they'd been created to find the light.

3.

The retreat coincided with Ramadan, so I happened to be fasting. I was relieved to find that another woman was fasting too. We smiled at each other across the table at afternoon tea. Then there was yoga. I'd never done yoga before. 'Focus on the breath. There is only the breath,' the yogi said in a European accent while I struggled into position. Ohmmm. I am no good at this. Pigeon, dog, snake. Ohmmm. 'Nothing but the universal breath.' Ohmmmm. I pushed myself into the poses as well as I could in a body that had been disconnected from breath for so long that it struggled to hold breath and pose at the same time.

When the sun went down, I broke my fast with a sip of cinnamon tea. Dinner was a vegan dish of eggplant curry served with a pink vegetable mash, rocket and sundried tomato. A white man with a shiny shaved head placed the meal before me with a slight bow, with a sort of care and humility that I had never witnessed before in a white man. He handled the bowl of curry, cupping it gently with both hands in a way that I have rarely seen men be gentle. *Had this been the norm, out there, perhaps there'd be fewer of us in here,* I thought. As he walked off, I noticed his feet were bare. He seemed happy, in a way that men rarely seem happy.

4.

I took my deluxe Scrabble board to the retreat with me. Four of us sat around the dinner table after everyone else had left: Linda, Linh and the other fasting woman whose name was Bintu. Bintu said her family was originally from Mali, but she'd migrated to Australia from France. A few turns into the Scrabble game, she protested in a French accent, 'It is not fair! English is my fourth language so I cannot compete with you all.' We decided to make the game equitable by allowing her to put down French words on the proviso that she did not trick us with any fakes.

This innovation restored the flow of the game. Bintu put down the word 'lac' and I asked her what it meant. 'Lac...as in, lake...as in, the water,' she explained. I tallied the score. Linh, whose parents fled the Vietnam war, said, 'Lac is a word in my language too, actually. It means "armpit".' We laughed. Linda, who is Lebanese like me, jumped in and said, 'Well it's a word for us too!' I frowned at her and said, 'I don't think it is,' to which she replied, 'Yes – lac shuuuuu cuz!' She drew out the *shu* like she was the biggest Leb in the area even though she went to a private school and worked at a top-tier law firm.

When we were done giggling, Linda pointed out that French words had entered Lebanese vernacular because Lebanon was once colonised by the French. Linh said, 'So was Vietnam!' and Bintu said, 'So was Mali!', and I said, 'Three different countries on three different continents but our homelands were all colonised by the French. So much in common!' We all laughed again, and the laughter subsided in sighs.

5.

The next day, a mental health professional in resort wear came to speak to us about breath. Not soft sighs or laughter, but the strenuous grunts associated with fury and vomit and childbirth. She taught us about engaging the parasympathetic nervous system by expelling breath upwards, from the diaphragm into the open. She explained trauma, the Kubler-Ross Grief Cycle, and the effects of stress on the body.

I sketched a diagram of the brain into my notebook as she spoke and labelled the key parts: thalamus, hippocampus, amygdala. Then I listed the various symptoms associated with stress: headaches, indigestion, mystery muscle aches. Brain disconnected from body. 'Perpetrators take joy in the disruption of connections between mother and child,' she said, and I wrote that down too. It validated something I had sensed for a long time. The disruption of connections. Disconnection. Brain disconnected from breath.

I added a final note to the bottom of the page: *Reconnect with breath.*

6.

That evening's activity built on some of the breathwork we'd been doing throughout the day, albeit in a less scientific way. One of the facilitators said that we would be taking a shamanic journey to meet a spirit animal or guide. I gave Linh side-eyes and she raised her eyebrows back at me cynically. I suppressed a laugh and told myself that I would be open-minded about the activity.

The facilitator consecrated the space with sage, dimmed the lights and began drumming. Boom, boom, boom. I exchanged a final eye-roll with each of my friends before settling back onto my floor pillow and closing my eyes. Boom, boom, boom. 'This is a deep meditation and you are completely in control,' the facilitator said. My breath began to rise and fall with the pace of the drum. Boom, boom, boom. 'You are walking in an open plain and there is a tree ahead of you. Walk towards it and you will see an opening, an entry. Step in and you will find yourself in a cave...' Despite my resistance and doubt and the urge to laugh, I descend into the cave. It is a dizzying, glistening space. I am tempted to open my eyes but I am too curious to leave just yet. Prompted by a now distant instruction, I sink into a chair carved from stone and furry creatures, big and small, begin passing by.

I meet a wolf. *How clichéd!* Some self-aware part of me is disappointed with my subconscious mind. I push aside thoughts of Instagram hippies and their tacky watercolour wolf artworks and try to get a better look at my wolf. It's handsome, with silky fur and serene eyes.

It walks and I follow. Then it runs and I follow, effortlessly. It urges me to run faster and faster and soon we are no longer in a cave; we are in a forest. The forest is woody and I am running with the athleticism of my body at twenty-one, the length of my hair at eighteen. My feet sync with the boom, boom, boom of the drum.

Flooded with breath, I run, and the wolf runs, and the voices of judgement and doubt recede as forest flashes by. The land I am running on reminds me of the hills of my parents' homeland. I run to a border and gaze into the occupied space beyond it and then I run back in the other direction to a castle or a palace or perhaps a shrine. A shrine of silver and green. A shrine in a little clearing in the woods. I pause and run my fingers over the silver lattice with which the shrine is decorated. I run some more with my wolf, who only slows down when we reach a stream. The stream is cool and clear and I enter it, waist-deep. Breath is so easy in this realm. Rinse, breathe, rinse, breathe. My wolf watches from the banks of the stream. I step out, rejuvenated, and notice a light behind my wolf. The light grows and glows and swells into form, into a figure with the outline of a person made of nothing but light. It steps out from behind my wolf and I cannot stop staring at it. It's as white as the sun but I cannot lower my gaze. We behold each other for a moment and then the figure dissolves. It dissolves into a cloud of static and glitter and sand. The tiny particles drift into the air in a single funnel and the funnel bends in my direction. It extends, narrows and shoots towards me in a fine strand. Like a golden thread entering the eye of a needle, the string of light particles enters my eye. It pours from the air right into my pupil and my pupil welcomes it, consumes it until there is nothing left of the shiny, glowing figure. Until I have completely unseen it. Until the beat of the drum changes, calling me back.

7.

The next morning, I woke up before sunrise for my suhur, which was a swig of water and two Panadols – the type with the caffeine in them. This is a hack I use to counter the caffeine withdrawals I sometimes get in Ramadan. Then I prepared for my fajr prayer. I'd fallen out of the habit of doing this, but figured this retreat, this Ramadan, would be a chance to recommit. I moved quietly through the blue-black air of the room I was sharing with Linda, wiped my head, arms and feet with water and prayed, slowly and deliberately.

At home, my mind had struggled to fall quiet at prayer time, but this retreat was still enough and dim enough, to experience 'It'. The calm I had been seeking. In Arabic, it is called *Khushu*: to pray with undivided attention, from the spirit. I pulled all my focus towards breath. The breath of my friend sleeping nearby. The breath of the morning outside, rustling leaves and jingling distant windchimes, which made me think of a pattern found in Islamic art called Breath of The Divine, a geometric pattern representing the expansion and contraction of breath, the oneness in many. The breath of a frog ribbiting just outside our door, which made me think of buccal respiration, the way a frog adjusts its breathing so that it can have breath whether in water or on land.

My breath. Deep breath. Inhaling as I stand, exhaling on *sujood*. Feel the grain of the wooden floor against my forehead and palms. The breath of me, warming the ground in front of my face. Holding breath, holding pose. Brain reconnecting with body, reconnecting with breath.

time lapse

Olivia Hamilton

hey have you

                um

what was I saying?
there's a thing –
a thing I need to –
what's that?   you need to leave?
oh sure   sorry   have a great day!
now where did I put

            um

why am I in this room
again?
keys...   no, not now, now is...   food?
no – work!
but did I eat already?
not food – work!
only fifteen   browser tabs open   that's not so   bad
check emails but wait –
dog barking   better let him in   side
pat the dog   (happy place)
wait –
I'm supposed to be –
ok, work
read the same para   graph   five times
still   don't know   what it   says
I'm hungry
did I forget to eat again?
shit
late for a meeting
ok, zoom   then food
read that paragraph again
oh, you're home.

hey have you seen my –

sorry   I mean   hi, honey   how was your day?

how was mine?

um

walk the dog

then couch –

but wasn't there   something –

something I was meant to –

Thank Christ I'm Not An Altar Boy: (Marist College Canberra 1975 to 1983) – for the survivors

Lajos Hamers

nothing's gonna touch you in these golden years
David Bowie, 'Golden Years', 1975

caps & bare legs, blazers & ties
bruised knees, genuflect, signs of the cross
a communion, a confirmation, an initiation
never changed socks – the smell of the corridor
cane Cain, Abel to cane Cain, cane Cain (only the best will do)

race for the cricket nets, slow down in the corridor
model plane wars, football cards
sultana sandwiches, salami sandwiches
it's reffo sandwiches for all

mum & dad asunder, papa put under the daisies
my left eye left leaning can't spot the ball
scrape and stitch – a deadman's eye
(what a trip at 11 – waiting for the donor to die)

teacher's nervous breakdown
she's caning in alphabetical order
'Louis is bone lazy' (but quick enough to flee at D)
white cassocks & black cinctures – it's a black noose
in cowboy films the good guys wear white
one bad apple, unlike Eve, unnoticed

> suscipiat Dominus sacrificium de manibus tuis
> [may the Lord accept this sacrifice at your hands]

moving on up
long pants, no caps, blazers & ties
genuflection & crossing, signs & bent knees
socks need their washing & faces need bathing
too big for the cane but they know you're still able

football every weekend, punches for communism
teachers to drool over, girls & their funbags
take a little wine, then take a little more & a little more
& a little more

parents kaput
dead-shits on ice – 'god your mother can pick-em'
left eye still stinging, the dead man wants out

another nervous breakdown, close to home
dial triple 0, hold onto mum's hand
white cassocks are circling, weighing up your worth
I think to myself, 'I've never seen The Birds'

ad laudem et gloriam nominis sui
[to the praise and glory of His name]

college years arrive, same blazer, new tie
the shaping of young men, in 'voluntary' religious devotion
clothes + hair, more than just things to wear
no cane anymore, it's purely psychological

sport, sport, sport & music
girls turn into women – not a fucking clue
first joint, first bands, first sex (not yet)
hang out, act cool & try to figure out what the hell to do

the family is under ambulatory care, our paths are here & there
it's a cock-eyed world & nothing is clear

the breakdown becomes personal
they were hiding in the halls
the statute of limitations is a life raft (for some)

                              ad utilitatem quoque nostram,
                         totiusque ecclesiae suae sanctae
               [for our good and the good of all His Holy Church]
                     run for the shadows in these golden years

Balancing Act

Maddie Godfrey

there is a tightrope in my kitchen that nobody else can see. made from thread that shines like spider web. yet even when I clamber, clutch at cupboards, beg to break the lineage, it will not untether itself. my love, much taller than me, bangs their head on the thread and it does not constrict around their brain. their bowl stays the same size. not ocean, not lake, just a ceramic circumference that hasn't changed since yesterday. I walk for hours at my favourite park, the footpath like an infinity loop on Tumblr's teenage wrist. there is no achievement in repeating the same routine until the ache relocates from your mind to your hips, but there is sustenance in repetition. once, controlling my illness meant controlling my mouth. now I know that even streetlights feel hunger. I do not mention the tightrope to my mother. still, she flinches when she opens the fridge and silver thread shudders above. my father delivers Tupperware containers stocked with soft landings. my recovering body

a balancing act. starvation is an imaginary friend I am grieving. my smallness; a sequence of stick-figures engraved on splashback tiles. before bed, I lay on the kitchen floor staring upwards. the tightrope, tangled into a loop, stares back: a shard of mirror stretched too thin to see myself in.

Notes for my newly dead

Rachael Wenona Guy

Hair is not something you need when you are dead.
Opinions, wit and clean fingernails will get you nowhere.
Lips are not desirable, beauty is meaningless.
Your high-domed cheekbones and ample bosom have no currency now.
Eyes are redundant, the emptied shells of your ears hold no music.

Perhaps death is like an infinite dormitory,
you are the new girl on ward.
Here, everyone is allocated the same elemental bed,
no preferential treatment is given.
There will be no whispering at lights out.
No one will steal from your locker.

Uniform is standard issue – memory, humus, dust.
The rations are identical – *Here, take this cup of nothingness,*
this empty bowl. Give me your remnant hunger, your erased wanting.
So many unquenchable tongues –
all turned to ash.

Death dries her wings by the river

Rachael Wenona Guy

2019 digital drawing

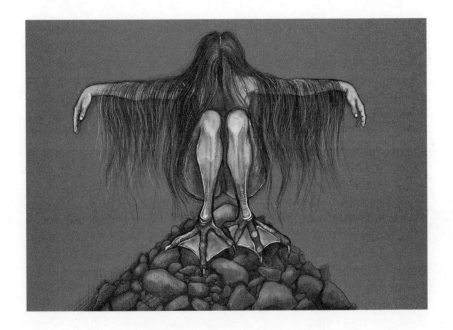

Once in a lifetime (job)

Andrew Galan

Stephen Hawking, Terry Eagleton and David Byrne meet me at my
building's front door
>One.

You may ask me,
>what these things are

I may tell you,
>I don't know

'Entropy is a measurement of disorder'
>Two.

Lack of order or predictability; gradual decline into disorder
My favourite job involved reading short but multitudinous
paragraphs about people doing things and planning things, and once I
had read enough paragraphs about people doing things and planning
things, I wrote a paragraph of one hundred words about the people
and the things they did or planned in those paragraphs, or specific
paragraph or selected grouping of paragraphs. The audience loved it.
It was an exclusive audience.
>One.

My exhaustion is inexplicable. I eat groceries. Go places. See films.
Visit the city. Read books. Watch programs. Wear clothes. Go other
places. Take pictures. Get sick. Get Well. Be attracted. Be attractive.
Do work. Ignore work. Make money. Spend money. Make my bed.
Sleep. Wake
up.
>Two.

These paragraphs about people and the things they did and planned
would build upon each other for weeks sometimes months until I was
expected to write something longer than that paragraph. If the timing
was right, I would put Talking Heads on my Dick Smith mp3 player
and to Life During Wartime I would get it done.
Often, when I drink enough coffee I fall asleep

Often, when I get out of the lift I forget which way to go
Often, I forget
'How, the reader wonders, can the evening look like an anaesthetised
body?'
When I forget why I sat down
'It is pointless to speculate about the existence of an "objective".'
When I forget
'There is no longer a grand narrative of progress
just a random collision
in which the present is
irreparable.'
     Three.
I thought if I went to the food court and ate
I might assimilate the viewpoint of the food court

St John's Wort

Alan Fyfe

A pinching wind will sting your face; while waiting for the pot to
boil; until it's dry and starts to burn; and when it burns you'll wonder
why; you set the pot to boil at all; you won't remember what good
food; you dreamed up when you started out; it must have been a
butter crumb; it must have been a homely smell; it must have meant a
time to sit; and edit half your yesterdays.

The wind's still going hard and high; the pot's still reeking from the
burn; you're hearing distant Wu Tang Clan; remember losing time on
that; you left the lost-times in the grass; ten years ago or maybe more;
and now it's more a brittle thing; a stem dried wholly to the core.

You'll say it's just like St John's Wort; a class A weed you kill at work;
it clogs up every nature strip; and bears up proudly in the drought;
still you asked around to find; the stuff's put to some decent use; the
herb's been tested double blind; and double blind was blind enough;
to feed the black-dog off to sleep; and thin the plump suburban
shame; a strong green life that thrives alone; and never begs a
gardener's touch; so happiness grows everywhere; and everywhere
we fight it off.

Brief intro to Benjamin Frater's poem 'The Argument'

Alise Blayney

I first met Ben at the University of Wollongong in 2005 during a creative writing class, and we were formally introduced by Alan Wearne afterwards. Such a twin flame meeting felt preordained and painted with poetry under The Pleiades, as we quickly became inseparable until his tragic passing in 2007.

Poetry was everything to Ben and, apart from his lived experience of schizophrenia, his whole identity. We always agreed that no matter what happened, poetry would be the bottom line, and that was exactly how we lived. I remember him saying at his dad's hotel, 'we're gonna eat, breathe, live, shit, piss and bleed poetry!'

Poetry was Ben's religion, medicine and emotional regulation, a powerful tincture and self-care elixir. Seeing that he saw the poet as priest, 'The Argument' is indeed a poem of both 'confession and exorcism' (by his own description). He believed this poem to be an incantation and grand grimoire about his lived experience and exorcism of psychic distress.

Much of the poem was written while Ben was admitted multiple times to what he referred to as the 'Bughouse', or Banks House, a psychiatric facility in Sydney's southwestern suburb of Bankstown. 'The Argument' contains an abundance of references to his time there, and is evidence of the profound shadow work he was undergoing.

Ben often said that his experiences of schizophrenia helped fuel his writing. He said it was a blessing and a curse that God gave him the whip of schizophrenia and the gift to write poetry. He was excavating psychic pain and transforming it into alchemic power and sorcery, navigating his own magic system through what he called a 'visionary poetics'. Such love and devotion to the craft allowed him to navigate and explore spiritual emergencies, mystical experiences and metanoiac voyages through these extraordinary seer-like states.

Ben was able to transform his scars into stars through the use of alchemic word thaumaturgy, and translate it into a form of schizoaffective logomania, in which he deemed 'a schizophrenic vernacular'. He conveyed to me that the repetition of the lines 'My forearm' were metaphors for 'self-harm', granting him poetic licence to explore his subconscious and transpersonal crises. The last lines of the poem 'living memory of BLEEDING VEINS AND BEATING WINGS!' suggests the release of distress through non-suicidal injury, signifying the paradox of trauma and catharsis.

Ben used poetry as pedagogy throughout his performances, and his poems were forever belted out with such high velocity that they felt like acts of ritual magic, creating a psychic charge so intense it transferred and was absorbed into the audience, jolting the nerves. You could literally feel his 'electricity shoved down the blue throat' going right through you, as though you'd been hit by a thunderstruck lightning of rapid-fire. Watching Ben perform was akin to experiencing what Jung called a 'Catalytic Exteriorisation Phenomenon', in which the psychic charge projected is so powerful that it causes external change in the real world.

I was lucky enough to see him do exactly that during his performance of 'The Argument' at a MAD Pride Concert at Campbelltown Arts Centre in 2006. We are also lucky that his performance was filmed and the footage can be found online. May Ben's rhapsodic force be with you and I hope you relish and revel in his electroshock rock as much as I do!

The Argument
Benjamin Frater

the dreamer who butchered his arm to challenge his reality,
now butchers his reality to challenge his arm.

My forearm is a wounded shark
My forearm is a crippled highway
My forearm is an imaginary tool
My forearm is a Nocturnal ballad of hieroglyphs,
        a battered-birdwing,
        a supplicatory of bleeding ghosts,
        the end of a lion's tyranny,
        an ancient Crocodile skull,
        the nightmare and war of Spring,
        a Catholic Yak's exorcism,

My forearm is our Golden fingerless child
        a piece of Apocalyptic debris,
My forearm has closed eyelids,
        is an Anti-american-warcraft,
        the memory of wild horses,
        its own executioner,

My forearm is Hell's kiss of smothered lips,
  your lack of perception
  the rage of a Blind Salamander,
  a voyeur while I sleep,
  a breast-less woman
  and a toothless old man tapping his foot to the
  rhythmic convulsions of a
  dead ocean,

My forearm is the active desires of Akhenaton,
  the left wing of Christ, the right fist of Allah
  and a Sanskrit-stitch-path,

My forearm is the bloodblack-Sunrise,
  a dead man's trepidation, a dread man's trepidation,

My forearm is A Subaqueous Prison,
  the mind that eats your leg,

My forearm is tomorrow's bitch, today's whore and last night's insomniac,
My forearm is a multitude of trenches and razor wire fences with the flesh
  STILL HANGING ON!

My forearm: a Luna ladder,
  a gutted reptile,

My forearm forces electricity down the blue throat,
My forearm is an arrow dreamt beyond this cell,
  a Chinese Red Rhapsody,
  an African Gunrunner,
  an Alcoholic automobile,

My forearm is an Aborigine wounded by the white FleshFlash of numerous
    Endeavours,

My forearm is our unclear nuclear future,
My forearm bleeds its own delight
My forearm refuses to bomb its enemies and dives into the rubble
My forearm is a solar backlash
My forearm invites refugees, provides none but exists in asylum
My forearm is the culmination of Hissing Apples and rotten skin,
My forearm is a docile blonde occupational therapist
My forearm is an Alcibiadian: the father of Flagellation
My forearm: a Hysterical Spartan Junkie
My forearm includes four thousand, seven hundred and eighty one billion,
    seven hundred and ten million, four thousand four hundred
    and twenty two Tentacles and as many years of Marineric
    tradition,

My forearm breathes through incisions also known as gills
My forearm is Marvell's dog,
    a bashed cherub,
    a thick vibrating web of Agony,
My forearm is a headless cemetery of flesh,
    affected by a 205 year old poet,
My forearm is a liar and tomb; a Miltonian Mutiny that groans t'ward
    the heavens,
My forearm is the unfurled Dragon abdomen with its five heads of
    blood and gristle,

My forearm remains remorseless for its mutilation

My forearm belongs to nobody

My forearm is a cut worm and blind maggot,

My forearm is a desperate corpse and Rabid carcass

My forearm desires the God of panicked birds and difficult Pyramids

My forearm is a sleepless cannibal,

My forearm is a liturgy of psychotic hooks displacing my mental weight
and suspends me nowhere in imagination,

My forearm is a meek neck waiting for the last train; our long red guillotine

My forearm bares the burden of backyard industry and institution,

My forearm witnessed the locusts under Paul's eyelids

My forearm can't wait for the gun to become a Mushroom

My forearm depicts a dappled sky and sickly horizon

My forearm will inoculate your reams of dreams

My forearm leaves your clitorial gland Yowling!

My forearm requires "more legs!"

My forearm remains defiant in the face of C.B.T and E.C.T

My forearm cannot lose or loose this RAW–Shackle

My forearm is a pillar of assassination and Masturbation

My forearm is a burning song-stick,

My forearm is Wracked and demented with Seraphic sinew;
the exalted Koala-Gut,

My forearm is a preter-mortem-Islamic-nocturne,
a bulging dead foetus,
a legless Noctambulist,
a deformed tiger eye,

My forearm releases its ghost in gaseous-dead-dove
My forearm is a syntactical activist
My forearm eats its own sores and admires the half baked moon
My forearm sleeps on rubber pillows,
My forearm is my brother
My forearm is a Kangaroo Blood Cult
My forearm is my mad hairless dog
My forearm exposes limp wrists to solar blades – My RA executioner –
My forearm observes the bomb-hollowed-world holding hopeless
candles, invites the world's collective Terror into its veins, up
arterial trenches, perforates my soul and shakes fire between
trembling scales,

My forearm stinks of Shark-Cunt, feels underbelly stingray sex, withholds
moray Eel masturbation and all the corporeal grandeur of
Marineric Mating

My forearm is the chant of a dead Nun, a tortured priest and dying lama
My forearm is the impure amazement and living memory of BLEEDING VEINS
AND BEATING WINGS!

dissociate is to

Helena Fox

Dissociate
is to separate
is to alter
is to leave

Imagine your particles
(your particular self), imagine
you are driving
a while or only minutes
in a car on a road with your children

Two hands/one wheel/thinking of
nothing/possibly Everything,
you feel the old pull out of your body, a tiny
snick, and you've shucked your skin

Now you are above the car,
you are rising, you have gone beyond the atmosphere
and reached, with no help from any science, the other side of the
universe

(Please understand, please feel this: the
space where bliss is waiting)

Dissociate
is to apparate
is to appear
is to arrive

In the car your son is telling you a story
or your daughter is telling you a story or
both of them are telling you a story

You do not understand them, they do not understand:
you are not here

You are driving
/ you are not driving
you are on the free   way
(and   you are n't)

Dissociate
is to disassemble
is for language to end
is for words to turn to water

•

Note:
People who are driving on freeways but also aren't
might forget they are driving on a freeway

You are on a freeway (with your children)
with your children
(alarms sound in the faraway)

You must come back

You must force yourself into yourself, stuff
yourself into your skin (what skin), rattle
back inside those bones (what bones)
return your farflung molecules, the ones that have turned
to air

Please do it

so you can take your children down this freeway past
these hurtle monsters
groan stone barriers
zipthick whitelines
all this gaping nothing—
and safely home

You walk through the door again
as you do
as you do

Keys clunk on kitchen bench, footsteps on tiles, cat snakes through
bare legs, mango sheen in sunlit bowl, dog wags at the sliding glass
window

Somewhere, someone moves through spacetime

Someone (a child) reaches out,
takes their mother's hand

Sweaty fingers, sweet press of
skin, here
here—

                                                    Here you are.

Paper Skin Cells
Ela Fornalska

I come from a cold
dark winter

My name is fire
known also as now
otherwise known as
crackles in the night

Yesterday I was doubt
also known as yeah... but...

Secretly I am sadness
known also as why

Tomorrow I will be enough
because today, I already am

From a cold dark winter
I came

I come from
Eggs in Concentration

From deep in my diaphragm
a voice comes through my larynx
green lungs breathe recovery

I live in many places at the same time

I come from stories and erased memories
I have inherited these unwritten poems
and hyperLINKs – hyper, hypo, hypersensitive

I have come from the BRINK of
death, depression, starvation, deprivation

I've learnt resilience
earnt empathy

The power of breaking

I am a yolk

Can I be a humble servant
collecting nectar in service
if freedom is a harness?

I gather pollen
and fill homemade
hexagons
with poems of
honey

I am the dawn
of my understanding
under this sun
I lie on the page
underneath my own pen

Cast off the knitting
I slip off these
needles and wrap
a clinging scarf
around my naked
neck

I am an empty field –
holding my solitude
is company enough
my code need not be broken

An internal red river
is setting diamonds alight –
alive

The paper knows better
than my pen, this storm
holding down a hurricane
muscles melt

I press play on memory
amplify olfactory

These thin slices of wood
absorb my heat

If burnt nothing is lost –
stored in my hippocampus
I hoard stories and collect music

I rewrite myself
over and over
it's the same journal
these pages
replace themselves like
skin cells

I press down the keys
type me up
it's tap tap tap tap soooooothing

The last time my therapist smashed everything I know about myself into ruins

Es Foong

I tell Phil, she's done it again.
Left everything in ruins, my eyes peeking
over broken piles of bricks, a crow
circling overhead looking for the birdbath
I put in the last time I had to rebuild
myself from ground up. It was a wrecking
ball this time, but at least she left
foundations. Time before that,

even the footings had been ripped
up, every rooted memory I'd used
to stand up my home was found
out, the neon nightmare of every room
in the house locked from the outside,
the percussion of palm
on cheek, the perfect pitch of broken
glass whistling inches from teeth.

Nothing to be done but build
again, this time a palace, this time
a home, a different set of histories
muddled, beige and green. Try
Lego, Phil says, try a spaceship,
try an artist's studio, try a hideout
for a motorcycle gang. But I root
around in the rubble, and there's

something under here
I won't let go.

Train Therapy

Michael Farrell

Pick a year, you would find me in tears if you found me, drawing on the train, through the fields, into Dubbo my comprehensible home. But pick a year, the reasons would keep changing. My head turned to face the strange wheat – green or languishing with drought; harvested. Maybe I was homesick, maybe yearning after someone, or mournfully thinking of the cost, of the profits of white bread. But these reasons –

These feelings – were only pretexts. If I had thought of fish instead, fish in blue, green, brown water, well, the release of the sympathy ducts would be on. I would be wishing the fields could be flooded. Probably I should have trained in and out for days, until I dried up. Then I would stop thinking the wheat was strange: their colouration, bending, sprouting, devastation, becoming integrated with whatever

Else I saw behind my eyes. I can't think of the town and the journey together. I could live on a train and drink bad tea for weeks, perhaps months. Every setback with a human, I could say to myself, 'it's good for your novel'. Every donkey, unicorn, blue devil, I saw munching through the window, every pterodactyl, or archaeopteryx, I saw circling above, or sitting straight up in the wheat: daring me to unsee them.

Fire Check Done/Room Vacant

Michael Farrell

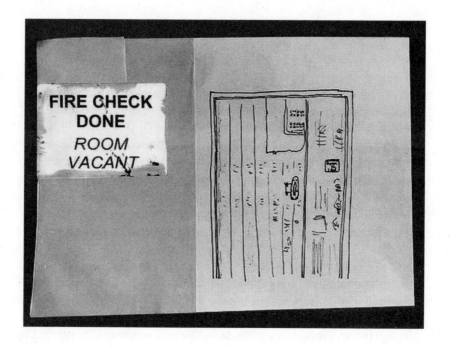

Hon. Crazie Ship

Heidi Everett

May I have your attention please.

Doors will be shut in ten seconds.

Stand clear.

Schizophrenia.

Throw all the letters in the air of Schizophrenia and it comes back down as Hon. Crazie Ship.

It's a ship that's both honourable and crazy.

It sank in flying colours.

HON 'An honorific is a title that conveys esteem, courtesy, or respect for position or rank when used in addressing or referring to a person' www.en.wikipedia.org/wiki/Honorific

CRAZY 'Someone who is wild and fun. Someone who will go against the rules. Someone who does what they want no matter the consequences. Someone who will do anything especially for love' www.urbandictionary.com/define.php?term=Crazy

Someone who spells it crazie.

My injured brain is high latency – you speak to me in 5G and I'm buffering Morse. Yet my thoughts are up there with Musk.

Except; the meds.

The meds put a full. stop. On. My. Thoughts. And. You.
Oh. Look. A. Dog.

A Tesla with Seroquel additive.

It'd be great if we all learnt Auslan and moved tangibly through
our shared minds rather than stood like pillars with invisible sparks
coming off the top expecting everyone to catch fire.

Schizoaffective.

It's not a tad of schizophrenia that affects me as a GP once described
to my body trying to engineer listening.

AFFECTIVE DISORDER 'characterised by dramatic changes or
extremes of mood, including elevated, expansive, or irritable mood
with hyperactivity, pressured speech, and inflated self-esteem, or
dejected mood with disinterest in life, sleep disturbance, agitation,
and feelings of worthlessness or guilt episodes, and often
combinations'
www.britannica.com/science/affective-disorder

Amazing!
Exquisitely spectacular phantasm of hypersensitive audiation.
What did you say?!
OMG a Dog!
...thing with   end   up front eyes?
Creative genius I
But I suck
the world sucks
This 3AM revelation
Enrages the crap outta me
a useless, discarded lump
fault.

All aboard.

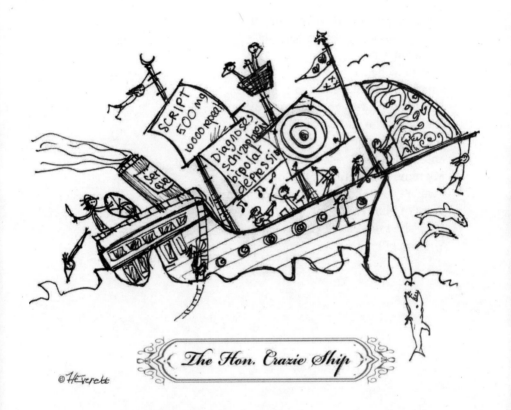

The Hon. Crazie Ship

© HEverett

Pear of Anguish

Gabrielle Everall

The man outside the seven eleven
shouted about my beautiful hair
Get a haircut
then he yelled
And lose weight ya fat moll
He kept repeating this over and over
It was as if he had placed
the pear of anguish inside my body
and turned the screw with his gaze
My mind was so full of this bondage
I wasn't sure I could love another woman
Least of all myself
Until she said: I'll kill your rapist
You can kill mine.

PTSD

Ali Cobby Eckermann

hey Man you wanna talk about ptsd

stricken prone in bed with anxiety
day after day and you hover nearby
always so ready to offer your cock

when the house is quiet in the city
wailing returns like a sea of desert
it's exhaustive and all I have from home

remarks at my mental health are cruel
none can measure my attempt to survive
the only solution in my mind is suicide

the need to isolate is so brutally intense
your offer to join me is not the answer
I love you and yet I must leave you now

blame my ptsd to console your grief
the anger you hold is for your mother
the removal from my mother is my trauma

hey Australia you wanna talk about ptsd

these notes they slip

Quinn Eades

we are mad to write and mad to not write we carry this book for
so long that it is become

                              un bearable

    in that we can not bear it, this doubling
                         tripling
                         quadrillioning of golden knife sharp
points and threads of light this collaboration of black holes this
battering at the self that is the command to write to lay down each
connection to follow the jumps

    I ask A *am I manic I think I might be manic am I*
        manic
    and A says that I am
    not and I ask *how do you know*
    that I am

                         jumping

                all o
    ver the place the

                         re are patterns in every thing I am   *awake*
and bright my in sides are a million refracted suns and this book
this book is falling   *into me into my body and I think I am*
manic
    and A says they know I
    am not I ask *how do you*
    know they say because when I am manic they can't follow
    my threads   and connections   they are tangled in
                my words   my insistent world making
                what I am saying all ways but they can follow this

so we make notes because we are not-writing and we are no-to-writing and the notes are on the backs of bills and scrunched along the sides of receipts and torn envelopes and we lose these notes they slip under the couch between the pages of books inside cupboards they make their own way and we are shattering we can't hold this many patterns these trillion ways of seeing these notes are important these notes keep leaving us it is all ways too much this vibrating these high screams resonances scintillations we are in ecstasy we are terrified a medieval mystic a rocking a shining open body we are given writing in the night in the down in the cup the well the tunnel we are filled with it

we are mad to write because writing tears us a part and we are tired of breaking of breaking our selves open on the cliff face of falling of hoping the up draft finds us this time again time again the down up the push of a great wind a cradle a supple rush all of a sudden knowing sky we are mad we are fucking mad to write we carry this book for so long that it is become

un bearable

in that we can not bear it, this bleating from all sides all corners under
grounds all ever y w here in that to bear means we carry a burden
means writing is a burden a weight a grinding down a suicide a laying down of arms a way of walking that says this insolvent state this way of being inside a cotton constant a fug of depression is how this life goes and we know with every thing in us that this is not ever the case it is the story the story of poets gone mad and see through in the night it is the romance of a creative life that is only also ever a tortured a short a desperate life but this is not how it feels to bear writing
writing is not a weight a rock in the belly the way stone tastes on the in sides a granite residue a cold middle a slowness a sandstone struck tongue a grief no

to bear writing is to inhabit a billion trillion sparks dog in the sun his red collar paws stretched the taste of coffee the secret paths of possums made in the night figs chewed ragged by bats a fight a shaking a shaken hand a screen gleam the panic that comes with fingers on keys so much so much we are bearing so many words so many ways to meet to weft and weave to glimmer shift to dive to be borne all ways in this supple wind to dig in to go down to go across to be horizontal outspreading ginger human hybrid writing is a rhizome in the body trauma is a rhizome in the body pleasure is a rhizome in the body what is a rhizome it is a root system it is memory it is how we find each other in the body how we meet how we love how we

un bear
how we write how we are mad not to write here is the book here is the body here is home

Roller Coaster

Kristen Dunphy

My wife's cousin hands me yet another lasagna, covered in Glad Wrap. The freezer is bursting with these compassionate gestures from friends and family who don't know what else to do.

She gives me a searching look. Are you okay? she asks. I tell her I'm fine. No you're not, she says. World War III is breaking out in the bathtub. One child has flicked soap in the other's eye.

She fixes me with a resolute stare. I can tell you're not, she urges. I am too tired to argue –

Slaying the Invisible Enemy

Moving down the blue-carpeted corridor towards room 15...

...and find her. The woman I share my life with. The mother of our children – curled in a tight ball. Lost. I sit on the edge of the bed, rubbing my hand over her back.

Come on, no staring at walls I tell her and manage to get her to sit up. What's up? I ask her lightly, in defiance of her mood. She shakes her head and whispers...she can't do this. Can't do what? I ask. Her eyes are turned inward. She's fighting an enemy I can't see.

I am the slayer. I should be slaughtering the rabid monster that shakes her in its furious jaws.

I suggest the breathing techniques she's being taught in group sessions but this makes her angry.

She clutches at her hair and pulls. Hot tears. She can't do this, she shrieks. I take her hands. Hey, hey – that's enough. No more of that. She begs me to do something. Anything.

I am an armoured soldier, sword drawn, poised to fight. But I don't know where the battlefield is.

Our three-year-old daughter plays with Exercise Barbie on the carpet at home. She stops, thoughtful.

When will Mummy stop being sad? she asks me.

I tell her she's more than sad. She's sick. In the tummy? she asks. I try to explain. In the head. Tummy. Heart. Everywhere.

She considers this for a moment. Then: who's going to fix her? The doctor? With Mummy's help. Yes. Mummy and the doctor will fix her together.

I am the anchor. I will hold fast amid the storm that wants to sink this family.

Illusions of control

I've come armed with my little flip notebook that charts months of suggestions, opinions, directions, changes in medication and concerns.

The doctor looks pained. I cite the long list of 'side effects' of the new drug he's proposing. He gives me a condescending smile, then explains most of those side effects are rare. The drug companies need to have themselves covered from every possible angle.

I challenge the decision he's making to change my wife's medication, suggesting she's been through enough without adding more to her suffering. He's infuriatingly patient with me. He even compliments me on my use of a notebook.

As I get up to leave, he opens the door and quips that internet research is fast becoming a nightmare for doctors. Looking things up on Google tends to cause more problems than it solves.

Applying logic

She's sitting up. We can beat this thing, I insist. I hand her a hardcover blank book. Every time she has a negative thought, she needs to write it down and counter it with the opposite.

She stares at the luminous pink butterflies on the cover. I ask her what she's thinking about right now. Nothing. Come on, I urge her. Tell me exactly what you're thinking.

The book goes limp in her hands. She's tired and needs to sleep. She curls up, turns her head into the pillow. I urge her to trust me, go with me on this.

It won't work, she mutters, barely audible. I open the book for her, hand her a pen. Okay, write that down, I say. This won't work, she whispers.

She closes her eyes.

Hope

She's been invited to a big awards ceremony following her nomination for a prestigious arts prize. I'm surprised she's considering it. We discuss with the medical staff the pros and cons of her going to Melbourne for the event. It could be too much? Or it could be just what she needs.

She looks stunning in her electric blue dress. Like a stranger. Makeup, earrings.

Who is this person? As we negotiate the plane, the hotel, the myriad colleagues and celebrities, she's gaining confidence. I am witnessing a miracle.

She is dancing. Sparkling. Her movements are suddenly fluid. I know this woman. She has returned.

I wake in the hotel room to the sound of the toilet flushing. She is violently ill. Crying again. Sobbing.

We canvas the possibility that there was something in the food but we both know it's unlikely. The Invisible Enemy has returned. She can't get out of the bathroom. Terror has her in its grip. And it's not letting go.

Despair

I'm called in to the hospital for a meeting with the Psychiatrist who has moved her from a Category 2 to 3. She's been talking about suicide again. The three of us sit in a tiny, windowless office.

The Psychiatrist asks her if she has had any plans about how she would do it. She stares at the ground. Silent. She's thought about throwing herself under a car. Or driving somewhere remote and taking pills. An intense, dry heat claws at my throat. My heart falls through an infinity of darkness.

Suspicion

What happened? How can a spirit so wretched burst so suddenly back to life? This is mind over matter, surely. Perhaps all this time she's had herself and everyone else fooled.

If she can turn it around for an event, then why not for other reasons? For us? For herself? Is there something she's getting out of being sick?

I am an anchor. I sway but I do not move.

If she were to go ahead with any of these plans, the doctor tells her, it's likely to be very damaging to her children both in the short and the long term. Statistics show that the chances they too will commit suicide themselves would be far higher, since it's been demonstrated as a way out. Suicide runs in families.

She's not registering any of this. Her eyes are vacant. She's somewhere else.

I tuck her into her bed. She looks at me, tearful. She's sorry for what she said.

She's so sorry. She can't help it.

Temptation

Till death do us part. The words rolled off my tongue back then as though they were one. We didn't deconstruct them or analyse them. We rode into our marriage vows with blind, optimistic fervour.

Until Death: meaning we remain together until one of us is no longer living.

Us: meaning myself and the woman that I loved, adored, was consumed by.

The bottom line being 'there is no way out besides Death'.

But what is 'Death'? Is it when the heart stops beating?

The woman I married is no longer here. She is the ghost of her former self. An empty shell. Can I be bound to someone who's not there?

Confession

Her doctor nods, softening his voice. The illness has a life of its own. There is no logic to it. It goes up and down and up and down. But gradually – with your support – your wife will recover.

The sand below me is shifting. The current pulls hard.

I've tried everything, I insist. I can't help her, I tell him. I don't know how.

Maybe you should ask her, he says. Ask her how.

Faith

She considers the question.

Just tell me I'll get better.

I do. I have. You don't believe me.

I need you to believe it *for* me.

She reaches for my hand. Holds it tight, her mouth quivering, eyes full of the black horror stalking her mind.

Don't give up, she begs.

I look at her. The shell into which I must believe she will return.

On you? I whisper.

Never.

Ghost Song

Jonathan Dunk

Thought is a cancer of time: the heavens die in their
orbits, bored of revelation, but our stubborn bricks
cling to the dead utopias of pornographic day. Take
this bread of quilted mornings and nail it to the ironic
streetlights. Let our shutterstock houses to wonder
where the ghosts went. Uber dead gods to bet against
addiction. Spend three days sober and rise again:
obsession is honest and Marx lacks false consolations.
Read John Forbes: *the truth that doesn't set us free*. Ghosts
are economies of scale and three days is too long to be
awake. Take this pill and follow it to the belly of a
whale, don't pray, but wake to whichever sun scalps
the waiting-room wall. Reddit will mutter that a
helicopter circles your favourite suburb, take the
difference on the echo of faith: this city is a desert,
and time stops in each day. Our state regulated faces
are rimed with coal dust and thc as we drift and snag
on thickets of twisting metal. If you think about it
you'll wake into or from dissociation on a street of
citric Californian bungalows and children-less bikes.
Scrawled chalk minerals will invite you to stand and
count for something and the angels in their crass and
violent splendour will mockingly demand your papers.
Who among us can claim to be essential with a straight
face. Twilight is more often and abruptly broken, most
songs will be the end of something at dawn. Satan has
room for compassionate grounds and the roadbeds
will be cool and clear as fatuous clouds fondle their
chemtrails. Descartes had trouble with daemons
pulling levers: *I shall consider myself as not having hands or
eyes, or flesh, but as believing I have these things*. But mine

and I are cell mates: don't moralise – delusions can be
tender but the paranoid fuck missed the point because
the real killer will be time, and he should have written
I think that I've thought that I've thought that I've
thought and repeat when it hurts. Corvid songbirds
have souls unfortunately: mania can be a dance but
for months the catastrophe stumbles on without
glamour: I is an it and it's all there is, your lovers are
shopping lists. We come to dawn to speak with the
dead, and in a catacomb of curfewed streetlights you
meet the shadow of an intimate stranger, and break
guilt with them nailed on empty streets like Christ's
thieves, and which of us is penitent depends on no-
one looking. The implausible shapes of our ghosts riot
and chant in the streets, see them trading lacrimal
glands, waving the holes in their wrists, and moving
their lips when they talk. Behold our industrial saints
with negatively geared halos filigreed in Yves Klein
lithium. Our funereal billionaires will outlive the sun.
Let the dead bury the dead, someone must.

Learning

Shastra Deo

after Wim Delvoye, Tim (2006–08)

While he sits on a pedestal in a museum empty
of human longing, I am at my desk alone
before a great mirror, his body in thumbnail
atop every window, still as a photograph
or painting or stone. A torso lit
up, beheaded by dark. I want to be him: a back,
a body, a stillness, or an ambling uncanny with a door

closed behind me. But my poem isn't about that.
My poem is about how I am
thirty and the land is yawing. I am writing
a message I can neither finish
nor abandon. I see my own face
in the ink of his skin. The man says he sees himself
growing old on that plinth, but only
in summer, and I think about that sort of surety, that
certainty of living until the end
of your time, of not
wishing for car wrecks or an executioner's axe or

the high justice of floodwater
and flame, and I am thinking that
I want to be liked. I want to be seen. I want to sit in
my body with my empty hands
and wait, again, for spring. I am thinking
the world had something
to teach me

once

but I haven't learned it yet.

On the 4th carriage from Flagstaff, howling

Kristen de Kline

07. When the virus first hit, I posted: BRING ME CAFFEINE AND LOTS OF PEOPLE.

08. I wasn't worried about catching it.

19. The celebrity couple in *No Idea* talk about surviving their 'darkest days'.

21. My shrink says: 'You can choose how you respond to things'.

20. They hunker down in a five-million-dollar house in Byron Bay.

04. Some skank posts on Tony's feed: *Go fuck yourself you fucking dog you're a fucking coward ... junkie piece of shit!*

05. Why can't she spell?

73. I'm over this bloody virus.

22. We've stocked up on Jack Daniels and a slab of Peroni.

48. There was a sun somewhere
      And it was dead   and black   and gasping

81. Tony tweets: *Deadly purple H doing the rounds.*

18. On TV I count seven people carrying one large steel bin with fluorescent lime-green handles. The garbage collector said: *There's been a horrendous increase in the number of rats.*

13. It reminds me of AIDS. No one gave a shit about us then.

14. At Heaven they stopped mixing Cosmopolitans. The cops wore yellow rubber gloves when they cuffed us. Don't believe me? Google it.

82. Tony again: *It's lethal and Naloxone resistant.*

83. My shrink says: 'Give yourself permission to feel rotten'.

84. The uber driver asks: *Do you ever look a passenger in the eye and wonder if they are going to be your killer?*

65. I'm strong, but it's getting to me now.

10. And another tweet: *Please be careful.*

03. The dog is not my friend.

55. *Beware the colour purple.*

06. Don't sniff everything. This is meant to be a walk.

16. What's going to happen to all my Qantas points?

90. It's Bill Gates. He wants to implant microchips in everyone.

89. I'm on the 4th carriage from Flagstaff, howling. There are rats ricocheting off my coat jeans sneakers.

91. Sometimes I bite my lip. My shrink has a lazy eye and a tainted accent. Sometimes I can't stop talking.

92. My shrink says: 'Have you tried mindfulness?'

66. It's Bill Gates. I tell you. He wants to profit from making a vaccine.

05. *More than once I've awakened with tears running down my cheeks. I've had to think whether I was crying or it was involuntary drooling.*

06. I stole that stanza from Jenny Holzer.

33. That's the third black Merc I've spotted at the crack house. I wish they'd offer me some gear.

22. We're turning into werewolves.

02. Sometimes. I. can't. come. down.

Role Models

Kobie Dee

Somebody tell us bout the way we living,
some brothers dead and some are sent to prison,
when I was young you couldn't tell us different,
but then again you weren't in our position,
look into the eyes of a teen who's never had nothing,
smoking bongs and drinking mosey with the speaker pumping,
down the park 50 deep relocate to the beach
a hundred teens getting chased by them punk police
and it was all fun and games until these drugs came,
popping pills and sipping liquor till the sun came,
aint no body there to tell us from a man's view,
I was snorting coke and selling drugs like a man do,
at least that's what I thought,
I know that's not the way I was taught
but there's some things a single mother couldn't teach us of course,
I learnt my lesson from the street and nearly paid the price,
overdosing in the park it nearly took my life,
and now I'm watching a friend who's lost it all to ice,
thinking will he ever get away from smoking glass pipes,
now he's at the bottom, old friends forgot him,
tried to get away but every body tried to rob him,
weren't no body there to guide him he just copied what he seen,
followed all the older kids he turned into a fiend,
so now I stop and think about my message to these teens,
aint no role model here just a brother with a dream
I just want to see a change
And everybody's asking me to change,
I'm just trying to take away the pain,
everything that I was taught was in this bottle
all we know is what we see and we aint had no role models
Old scars with new ways to cope,

old ways smoke weed pills and coke,
long days my mum seen it the most,
I was thinking bout my neck in a rope that's why I can't go back,
glad I got my life on track now I can finally be the father that I never
    had,
I keep my mind on my money so we can never be broke
and all my time because I know how much she needs a dad,
in a position, these kids always need a person to listen,
always thought I was alone cause we aint had no pot to piss in,
I was 16 with big dreams of mad living,
no role models just older cousins that's drug dealing,
ice addicts and alcoholics in my building twenty thirty five that's
the place that I got my life visions,
all I know is I'm gone keep with the facts,
I changed my life and I aint never going back,
I've gotta be that role model
And everybody's asking me to change,
I'm just trying to take away the pain,
everything that I was taught was in this bottle
all we know is what we see and we aint had no role models

What is Night In The Woods about? A personal essay

Josie/Jocelyn Deane

A disassociating college student from a working class background
drops out of college and returns to her childhood
home/town. She is a bi cat; she/you are human with a body
of a bi cat. Everyone is a cat of some kind, I imagine
her/you saying. Her childhood
best friend is a blue crocodile furious at her/you
for returning. Her contemporary best friend
sucks dick, throws knives, is off his ADHD meds, is
a yellow fox. The world is resolving into shapes:
racist monuments, the nostalgic parade float housing
baby opossums she/you cultivate with pierogi, stolen
a child's face under her fists, a muddy polygon.
She/you fail to connect with the youth of America
despite being—she states—still a youth of America
she waxes lyrical re: the slogan 'NUKE POSSUM SPRINGS'
sprayed over a mural of departing industry and
spirit workers. She/you learn her grandpa removed
the teeth of bosses, fucked uncomfortably.
Everyone here, at one point, has wanted to nuke
their home, even when the jobs were good
the shapes good… She/you sleep-walk into God
thrice: as a janitor, as a translucent lion, as a black
dog, filling the void left between interstellar
spaces expanding, endlessly: a shape approximating
a colouring book mini-game, outside the lines
a slam poem read in the town library, a familiar
late night show she/you can watch with your ex-miner dad
too old to be a mall butcher, your closed mine returning
the chants of cultists that believe the black dog will
make the jobs/children stay put, shapes approximating
shapes. She/you walk with your church-receptionist

mum in the wheat-stalks. The talk is seasonal
with avoidance of the topic: why did you come
home love? How circular were your classes, exactly? Speak
to your dad, please, he's going through the old stuff.
Her/your attic is a mine. The game begins with a poem
you/she selects. You/she does the same
in Kentucky Route Zero, you remember, a game about
debt. You/she presses A A A A to
answer the mirror/screen, to disassociate/talk to your/her
     -   self , to double-jump down the stairs, to dress up
     for Halloween, a sword through your/her head, having
     not got her lines for the production, playing
     a swamp witch, simply repeating
     eeh he he hee. You can't remember the end-game.
     Are you/she resting
     on a couch, with her dear friends, having escaped
     the dog cultists? Are you/she at the bus-station/statue of some
     cop, talking to a janitor? Do your/her parents still
     need to put the house on the market? Do
     the shapes continue to resolve, on the title/credits? Was it
a dog, or a goat?

'But you don't *look* autistic.'

Aloma Davis

Recent estimates suggest that up to 25 per cent of women on the
autism spectrum are not diagnosed.

True, I am not a trainspotter,
a toddler lining up his dinosaur toys,
or a hand-flapping Dustin Hoffman boy.
I am another:
a confident woman, funny teacher,
loving wife and mother.

You are having a moment of
      c o g
            n i t i ve
d is so   n a n ce

I understand. You've been misled.
For you, I am like that reading test,
the one where the word 'blue' is written in red.

At this point, you're getting a little hand-flappy yourself.
'But you're not *autistic* autistic. We're all a little autistic, aren't we?
I mean, I don't eat peas!'
True. I, too, don't like peas.
But I had it confirmed by a psychiatrist
using the Diagnostic and Statistical Manual of Mental Disorders: V.
It doesn't mention peas. Curiously, it also doesn't mention trains.
Perhaps you should write and complain.

It refers to *Adverse responses to specific sounds or textures.*
'Ha! I've never seen you sit curled in a corner and rock.'
True. But have you ever seen me wearing socks?

It refers to *Deficits in social-emotional reciprocity.*
'But you make such good eye contact! You're so expressive!'
Yes. But if you ask me what I think of your new haircut,
I will literally tell you what I think of your new haircut
expressively, while making good eye contact.
Or would you rather ask me to *compliment* you on your new haircut?
Please be specific.

It refers to *Highly restricted, fixated interests that are abnormal in intensity or focus.*
'You don't memorise the train timetable, do you?'
Of course not. But give me a moment and I will tell you in lieu
about Eugene Schieffelin, a nineteenth-century gentleman who
introduced starlings to the United States. Did you know he released
first 60, then a further 40 into Central Park, New York? They now
number over 200 million. They should call him the 'Father of the
Starlings' but I think farmers call him...other epithets.

Oh look at that. I made you smile. That is a social cue to continue.

It is probably apocryphal, but they say his goal was to introduce all
the birds named in Shakespeare's works to the United States. I think
that's a noble goal. Environmentally catastrophic, yes, but noble. If it
had worked out, children would learn about him in textbooks and he
would have a global Netflix biopic made about him starring Jude Law.
Instead everyone despises him and I find it   unbearably sad.

Now you're giving me awkward silence and I don't know what to do
with that.

Perhaps I should tell you more about Shakespeare and birds.
Everyone likes Shakespeare, right?
Wrong.

I am a foreigner in your country.

You have different customs and bluntly
social faux pas follow me around.
People don't excuse them because
'I don't *look* autistic.'

But, like a foreigner,
please stop being surprised
when you realise
autistic people are just

people.

Surely now you see.
You're right.
I don't look autistic.
I look like

me.

Love Letter

Andrew Cox

I apologise
      To this body
           For calling it
           Such a   selfish vessel.

We will call this a love letter

For in this moment
      I will ask you to
           Forgive yourself.

           As i ask myself,

                        With this body laid bare

. Unhinge my lips
      . Unlock my jaw
           . See myself and say,
                I forgive you,
        Forgive the years of self hatred.

                Forgive what is not fully made,
                Maybe, never will be.

    This life   is more circle than line.
    We keep   growingandgrowingandgrowingand...

Forgive your skin.
      May still feel a sluggish suit.
           Hand-me-downs you have not yet grown into,

Although you will, won't you?
       have you not done timeandtime again?

The way you make the most of what you have,

  Spin something out of nothing,
      Spin some magic out of air.
             Survive / despite / in spite
             Of what want's you not to

Watch yourself c r u m b l e in the mirror
How a wave might   c r a s h

    Watch how far you've come,

                See / yourself
                Love / yourself
       Before, Anyone / else
                       Will.
                   ! You have to,

   this.*whisper*.will.be.more.*survival*.than.a.*scream*.could.ever.be

Motherlines

Radhiah Chowdhury

To the best of my knowledge, there's no term for 'mental illness' in the Bengali language. There's 'matha kharap', literally 'bad brain'. There's 'pagal', or 'crazy', the word I've heard used to describe any mentally ill unhoused people and also the pangs of longing and love. Less common is 'psychic', possibly a term specific to my extended family, who at some point heard and completely misunderstood the word 'psycho'.

The one that has stuck with me for decades is 'jinn dhorse', a mind that has been caught and possessed by a jinn. Given the Bengali penchant for telling terrifying but broadly plausible stories of possession to young children, the first time I heard the term used to describe my behaviour, I panicked. How was I supposed to go about getting *un*possessed? Most jinn stories we were told involved people making narrow escapes from malevolent spirits, not what to do once you'd done something so ill-advised as to *be* possessed.

My mother used the term most often, most often in reference to me, but never with any malice. More usually with despair, confusion. A young migrant mother in a country town with three small children understandably had very little wherewithal to comprehend that one of those children wasn't being noncompliant and destructive for shits and giggles. As I grew up and we moved to Sydney, the lines between the normal levels of teenage asshattery and whatever was going on in my head were blurred beyond recognition. That's when she started using the term with resignation. Four kids by that stage, a husband who worked overseas for long stretches, there was bound to be one rotten egg in the lot. Maa's reaction to any conflict is to retreat and shut down, and boy, did I give her plenty of conflict in those years.

My mental health journey can be traced along motherlines, fractals that continue repeating in subtly changing patterns across generations. As a young adult, I learned that my Nanu had lived with paranoid schizophrenia for decades. Untreated, of course – by the time she was my Nanu, age had lent her behaviour a benevolent eccentricity, but her journey was never a happy or smooth one and she met a premature and violent end that still wounds us nearly twenty years later. Maa was never able to comprehend her own mother. She treated her with varying degrees of anger, impatience and disappointment. Then Nanu was gone. Only a handful of months later, my diagnosis finally came in. I would have been nineteen, perhaps twenty. Maa banished Dad to the spare room and called me into her bed that night, and as we lay there in the dark, she held my hand very tightly and whispered, 'Don't tell anyone else about this.'

Counter to most of my upbringing, I obeyed Maa on this point for a very long time.

We didn't speak of my mental health or treatment after that night, not through the medicated years and the fug of assorted high-dosage SSRIs, nor through a number of episodes that broke through that fug. She almost broke her silence once, when my high school best friend, of whom she was incredibly fond, was admitted to an inpatient unit after an unsuccessful suicide attempt. She ended up channelling her fear and sorrow into making weekly batches of bhapa pitha for me to take for my friend on my visits.

When I recount that night in Maa's bed to others, her words are almost always met with a sense of horror and condemnation. It made me think about whether I should write this particular piece for weeks. I never tell the story to castigate my mother, or to showcase the ignorance of my cultural heritage on issues of mental health (I'll generalise that a version of this story exists in every single culture). The moment is crystallised in my memory not because of what Maa said, but because of the strength of her grip on my hand as she said it, as though by holding me firmly enough, my usually undemonstrative mother could haul me out of the pit that swallowed her own mother, two brothers and several nieces and nephews. That memory has always cut through the silences. That grip still holds firm even when the words can't be spoken.

Talking about feelings is not something Maa's ever done with ease. Her care and attention are always demonstrated via food and folded laundry and clean sheets. I learned that language; I'd like to think I'm fluent at it. My sister's grasp is more remedial, and she spends a lot of time being angry, impatient and disappointed that Maa doesn't react to our shifting mental health journeys in ways that she understands. She's a mother now herself, and a GP specialising in mental health. Her seven-year-old daughter has yet to be diagnosed, but we can recognise the signs that some mental health support will be needed at some point. A few years ago, Maa commented on how much my niece reminds her of me. She didn't look happy as she said it.

Versed as I am in Maa's silences, I have observed her closely in her dealings with my niece. The tightness of her grip is there in the way she teaches my niece needlecraft, just as she taught me decades ago back in that country town. The way she arranges to always have my niece's favourite manoush in the oven whenever she visits, and the many hilariously oversized outfits she sews for her. The way she has never said 'jinn dhorse' when my niece has acted out.

In our preliminary session, my first psych told me that I should think of treatment and recovery as a nonlinear path with an ever-shifting end point. 'We're going to approach this in terms of measurable, achievable goals,' he said. 'If we can see how things are changing, and hopefully improving, I think it'll make the next step that much more achievable. And we're going to keep working at that.' Despite the imperfect methodology, I've remembered that conversation at different points throughout the last twenty years, but most particularly when I think of the motherlines of my mental health. I can see how those fractals have changed, subtle, infinitesimal, but tangible, just as much as I can see how they remain the same, grounded in fear, uncertainty and love, always love.

There's no one word for 'love' in the Bengali language. A cursory google will reveal more than thirty words of varying nuance – 'prem', 'bhalobasha', 'doya', 'mamta'. I trawled through the ones I know, trying to find a suitable one to describe a mother's anchoring grip. I've never heard Maa tell us she loves us in as many words, not me, nor my siblings nor her grandchildren, neither in English nor in Bengali, so I don't have that as a reference. I've abandoned the search and instead relied on the language that Maa has taught me over thirty years. A steaming bhapa pitha, fresh from the pot. A collection of squares cut from all our childhood outfits, fashioned into a patchwork quilt for the grandchildren. A warm, strong hand holding firm in the dark.

The longest resident

Jen Chen

Was transferred when this ward first opened.

Regular routine, has a preferred seat.

Compliant, punctual, polite.

The voices do not tell him to hurt people,

just to sleep on his right side.

No friends or close relationships, no contact with children.

Wants to stay indefinitely.

Rehabilitation plateaued.

Bed blocker, a static patient.

Cries inappropriately.

As themselves (believed and seen)

Wendy Burton with Pascalle Burton

and so, people underestimate you?

yes.

I sat on a chair –
I was determined to find my Guide
I'd read a book on how to do it –
so I'm sitting on a chair just really straight and still
and then I felt my arms moving up—

[raises arms and grimaces because she has bursitis in her right shoulder]

seen and unseen

I closed my eyes and saw a pathway of cobblestones and an arched door. and I walked down the brick steps and went into a room and G – I didn't realise it was G at first – there was a man sitting with coat tails playing the piano. I decided this must be my Guide. and who do I know that plays a piano and is elegant enough to wear coat tails? Oh, of course, it's G!

and throughout our time on earth, he's cropped up so many times. he's just done so many nice things for me.

they tend to think schizophrenia is hearing voices or seeing something on TV that's talking just to me and I've never had that. I never once had that. and they said, 'you'll get it because you're schizophrenic.' and I didn't, I only got Calling In, which is totally different to having people talking in my ear.

describe Calling In.

I feel their presence throughout my whole body and if they've got something sore or something, I'll feel that. and if they want to go to the toilet and I've already just been, I have to go again.

seen and unseen

they don't know what mentally unwell or delusional actually looks like.

a hospital story:
I was in a ward and this girl had no clothes
so I gave her my only dress
and then not too long after she said to me,
'I'm going to kill you, you deserve to be murdered'
I went and hid in the lounge behind the chairs and went to sleep
then I heard the nurses saying, 'she's got to be somewhere.'

seen and unseen

haloperidol: the second it touched my body, I was stiff. absolutely stiff.

well I had 304 people in me and the doctors couldn't believe how far I'd counted them. I could speak to them. and then a whole lot of other ones came and they didn't belong and they weren't invited. so I made a really big brown paper bag. I was inside it and I closed it with staples. I could hear the other people in the ward and there was someone singing off-tune and there was a couple cracking jokes and I was safe because none of them could get in and it's not much of a story.

well I think it's a
great story.

a hospital story:
this girl was having a shower
she said, 'will you be my mother?'
and I said, 'yes, I can be your mother'
and she says, 'could you wash my back?'
so I'm halfway through washing her back and the nurse
came in and said, 'you get out of here! that's not the
done thing!'

believed and disbelieved

tardive dyskinesia:
Dr D said, 'you're
gonna have that
all your life.' but I
haven't, have I?

I had a little sentence I'd say to get
rid of them. I'd say, 'are you invited?
are you belonging?' and if they said,
'no,' I'd say, 'go back from whence
you came, never to return again. so
be it.' and that worked.

a hospital story:
there was a really nice guy visiting his wife and she
was really nice and he brought her a Dean Martin CD
collection with forty songs on it. and they were sitting at
a table listening to it. so me and my brown paper bag
went and sat down under the table to listen and I was a
bit snuggled up to her legs (she didn't mind). and I told H
that I'd really like a Dean Martin CD—

I helped H get it
but I didn't
know that's why
you wanted it.

I just
remembered. I
think I got that
Dean Martin
box set from
Sanity.

[they laugh]

clozapine, which was
so much better than

risperidone, which was
so much better than

haloperidol.

and the things that I experience,
though they might not be normal
to other people, they actually bring
me calm and peace, joy, play and
humour.

seen to be believed

I used to suffer shame but I don't
now. we've got beyond that.

yes.

IF I SMELL GAS AND THERE IS NO GAS or AM I A PSYCHOANALYST IF I DON'T HAVE A COUCH?

Pascalle Burton

Sure, we love the mad, but only if we ourselves get to decide the conditions for what the madness will look like.
Aase Berg[1]

I start horizontal on a worn, olive-coloured recliner. A cliché for an essay on mental health, except I'm here for my mouth. A few days earlier – where it really starts – I was reclining in my dentist's chair, complaining about my tongue. Since a drawn-out tooth-extraction-and-implant ordeal, I'd developed a persistent habit of sucking on my back left top teeth. It was bordering on obsessive, where my numb tongue's scything swipes were all I could think about, so my dentist recommended a hypnotherapist who could break the uncontrollable urge.

I wouldn't typically opt for hypnotherapy. Too many stories about therapists assaulting their patients. This one, who operates one floor up and a block away from my dentist, assures me that consent is key, that he will not touch me and that I will be 'present' throughout the sessions. His focus isn't on weight loss or regressive hypnosis, either, which sways me to give him a go. A part of me wonders if it is my evaluation or his aptitude that won me over.

Two reclining chairs in this piece already. They are icons typically associated with psychoanalysis. For Mark Gerald's project *In the Shadow of Freud's Couch*, he took portraits of fellow psychoanalysts in their offices; without fail, every subject had a couch. He recounts a senior New York analyst saying, 'I never use the couch with my patients, they always sit up. But if I didn't have a couch, I wouldn't feel like a psychoanalyst.'[2]

All this talk of Freud and couches makes me think about my mother.

I foreground this by saying that my mother is one of the sweetest people you could meet. She is gentle, caring and vulnerable and has a wacky sense of humour. And she lives with a diagnosis of late-onset schizophrenia. I grudgingly described her attributes just now – though I shouldn't have to – because, too often, her diagnosis influences how others relate to her. She knows when people treat her differently and understands it's their problem, but it can be demoralising. So it's easier to do the groundwork to combat stigma and to ensure she's regarded with respect upfront.

When Mum was first diagnosed, this was explained to a fifteen-year-old me as a chemical imbalance in her brain that distorted her sense of reality. Thirty years later, I understand that a chemistry approach to mental health is only part of the story, despite mainstream medicine being slow to catch on. Modern practice is trying to lean more towards including patients as participants, coordinating care in the community, and valuing a sense of self. However, Daniel Zola astutely suggests that 'the mainstream understanding of "mental health" creates much room for concerns centred around the loss of personhood, even as it views mental health as a problem to be managed'.[3]

I also need to establish that Mum has found ways to manage her mental health and has been stable for over a decade. This has not always been the case – she's had years of traumatic experiences that led her to where she is now. Today, she loves her current medication,* has a supportive team of doctors whom she trusts, works to minimise stress in her environment, and focuses on feeling calm and safe.

Mum also talks about it. She knows that she didn't choose schizophrenia, which has helped her shake off the forces of guilt. While nothing lasts forever, I understand how fortunate it is that these elements have been aligned for this long and that this doesn't always happen for people with a similar diagnosis. Institutional and policy reforms are certainly needed to address stressors and issues such as social and systemic discrimination, disadvantage, access, racism, fragmentation, misdiagnosis, marginalisation, punishment or exclusion. And sometimes, the drugs just don't work.

But consent matters. In the past, decisions were made for my mum without her consent. The narratives are tricky when psychosis and hospitalisation meet. There's the narrative about the psychotic episode where the goal is to stabilise. Then there's the narrative Mum's experiencing, which has other, mesmerising goals. She has been medicated against her will, given shock treatment and been the target of reverse psychology. On one occasion, our family had little choice but to section her. All devastating, and who could blame Mum for feeling paranoia and distrust in any of these circumstances?

Some of that medication caused very unpleasant side effects. In fact, Nathan Filer argues that *side effects* isn't quite right – rather, he says, effects that outweigh the drug's *desired effects* are really the *main effects*.[4] One *main effect* for Mum was *Tardive dyskinesia*, an uncontrollable movement of the tongue and lips. I ask my hypnotherapist – who is treating me for uncontrollable mouth movements – if he's ever treated people with schizophrenia. He explains that it requires their doctor's approval, but he's often worked with clients with schizophrenia to help them stop smoking. I nod, recalling the constant waft of tobacco in the psych wards where I'd visited Mum. A 2018 Cancer Council report states that 'people with schizophrenia are more than five times more likely to smoke than the general population, and tobacco-related conditions are responsible for about half of total deaths in people with schizophrenia'.[5] I've read that nicotine can temporarily counter or relieve psychiatric symptoms and, although there's no real consensus here,[6] I believe this form of self-medicating must offer some reprieve; otherwise, why would so many do it?

Mum doesn't smoke, never has. I did, for about fifteen years, but I chose to give up for my partner, a nonsmoker. I was lucky and never had trouble quitting, even though I loved smoking, especially cigars.**

There is one thing my mother does, though. She refers to it as Calling In. She describes it as feeling someone's presence throughout her whole body, including their emotions. When her Calling In is more frequent than usual, it can be a sign of an upcoming so-called psychotic episode. In the past, this has consisted of many extreme experiences, including feverish and sleepless Calling In sessions with a huge line-up of 'visitors'.

Calling In invokes an element of fear in me, I won't lie. I'm not concerned that Mum does it; in fact, I find it fascinating. But it's a behaviour that she, her GP, her psychologist, her psychiatrist and I monitor. My mother is extraordinary because she has learned that she doesn't need to be secretive about when and how often she Calls people In. But that is because she is supported to talk about it as much as she is supported in how she manages her own life.

What's wild is that I've started Calling In, almost every day since I started working from home during the pandemic. In online meetings, if we need to consult with someone else, we say, 'Let's call them in'. When it first happened, I got the shock of my life, but I've grown accustomed to the idea that something labelled delusional for my mother is a widely accepted practice in my working life.

Delusion and reality: what's the difference? Between reality and superstition? Between superstition and suspicion? Between suspicion and paranoia? Between delusion and psychosis? Between psychosis and clairvoyance?

I'm not convinced the lines are static or clearly definable. I'm not sure that my questions have discoverable answers. There's this part in Jane Dykema's 'What I Don't Tell My Students About "The Husband Stitch"' – a blistering, remarkable essay on belief and consent – that excavates something in me:

If I smell gas and there is no gas, am I different than if I smell gas and there is? Am I crazy, then, and does my value come from not being crazy? Does my value come from being right? If there is no gas, am I not right? Does it mean I didn't smell gas or does my experience of smelling gas still remain?[7]

Humans are often guided by some level of delusion or a loss of contact with reality. Like worrying. Worry can form an imaginary future – technically non-existent – and convince us this is useful for rational decision-making or problem-solving. When I was a kid, my bedtime had a specific routine because I was sure someone in the family was going to die overnight. So before I'd go to sleep, I'd say to everybody, 'See you in the morning!' in order to break the curse. And because it worked on the first night, I did it again and again.

Or trust. We constantly navigate situations where we make unsubstantiated decisions about who to trust and why or why not. How many times do we rub shoulders with delusions of reference, grandiosity, erotomania, erasure, nihilism or soma? Nathan Filer says, 'all people, including ostensibly "sane people", have a staggering capacity to believe in nonsense'.[8]

When a person – under the label of an artist – produces concepts that are nonsensical or original, the reflection they receive from their audience is encouragement, congratulations, light. For example, you can feel the energy in this tweet by Lidia Yuknavitch, a writer who has refused to 'follow the dictates of psychological realism':[9]

> When I see a shift in someone's art making over time I get really, really excited. Giddy. Breathless. I know exactly what I'm looking at/hearing/experiencing. I know they just risked everything and leapt.[10]

The recently departed musician and writer Greg Tate – whose writing 'froze and shattered time, supercharged neurons, unraveled familiar knots and tied up beautiful new ones'[11] – said that 'originality, like style, is generally what's left after artists eliminate all excess from their repertoire – all the corny stuff that seems better suited for someone else'.[12] There's nothing quite like consuming radical or unstable art that illuminates, transcends, liberates, radiates or mystifies. This sense of transformation reminds me of a line in James Hannaham's poem 'Knifemagnet':

> I saw myself as several things when someone saw only one
> and I used a word unknown to those outside.[13]

What is the line, then? Can my mother freely see herself as several things? When a person under the label of a psychiatric diagnosis produces original ideas, fear is reflected back at them. My mother has been discouraged from talking about her so-called delusions, but they are clearly a big part of her life. Why should she pretend they aren't happening? Is it to make others more comfortable? Is the fear that if she speaks her delusions into the air, they will multiply? To me, that concept is delusional.

If she speaks into the air, do we have to fear? What if we make space for the narratives of delusions instead of ignoring them or concealing them through shame? I love talking to Mum about her experiences. Sometimes her recollections are filled with exasperation at how far-fetched some of her past delusions were. These conversations feel like levitation because, in hindsight, she has unusual clarity about the line between her 'everyday' delusions and those that have required hospitalisation.

Joel Gold acknowledges that delusions are meaningful for a reason:

> Most of us take our own thoughts seriously and the basic premise of psychiatry is to think about thoughts. When we listen closely to what our patients are saying, paying attention to psychotic and non-psychotic thought with equal consideration, we foster the therapeutic alliance, and stronger alliances yield better therapeutic outcomes.[14]

Mum's psychologist is a perfect example of this. Without judgement, she invites Mum to talk about absolutely anything, and you can see the benefits. I ask Mum how that feels and she answers, 'It's such a relief. And the fact that you let me talk is an even bigger relief. If I know I can talk about anything then I'm open to love you as much as I want to.'

And that's it. These are acts of love. Intentional acts that the peerless bell hooks said mix 'care, affection, recognition, respect, commitment, and trust, as well as honest and open communication'. With love, says hooks, 'our fear may not go away, but it will not stand in the way'.[15] We can't navigate the future, but I hope that if we show her she's valued, Mum will feel open to share as often as she wants, again and again.

See you in the morning.

---

* After years of trying medications, Mum was considered 'treatment resistant' and invited to be involved in the high-risk trial for reintroducing Clozapine in Australia. As a result, she receives the drug free of charge. Dr Bessel van der Kolk was involved in the first test of this drug on chronic patients in the USA and describes the responses as 'miraculous'. See B. van der Kolk, *The Body Keeps the Score: Mind, Brain and Body in the Transformation of Trauma*, London: Penguin Random House, 2014, p 28.

** In case you need some form of closure, while Mum was told she'd have *Tardive dyskinesia* forever, she has defied that jinx. I also had positive outcomes from my hypnotherapy sessions: my habit of sucking my teeth decreased considerably and I also noticed a reduction in anxiety and chronic back pain. But I'm mindful that this is not an essay about endings and that things are in constant flux.

ON WAKING UP IN THE WARD AT OAKLEY

John Mukky Burke

mutterings and the mumblings
greying faces
I can't say vacant
that's been said before –
line up on their fence post bodies
like a tired linking string of rusted wire
and wait for blue ladies to bring
the breakfast evermore.
with the bucket – o – the yawning bucket
chucked half full with food half eaten.

but I won't be beaten
and at the pushing of the pills
for the very major ills
of – as they say – society –
that's me – so
I sit and eat marmalade and toast
and boast I'm not a piece of rusting wire
in need of galvanising.

afternoons of agonising
evenings filled with cards
some poor bastard
who can't play piano
though he tries so very hard.

the squeak of ordered sandals
the squeal of unearthed scandals
the flip flop flap of jandals;

then the pushing of the polisher
the same old tired demolisher.

*Opening 1867 in west Auckland as Avondale Mental Asylum,
the facility was renamed Oakley Psychiatric Hospital in 1960. It
functioned as this until its closure in 1992. Burke was a residential
patient on a number of occasions between 1973 and 1975. Jandals is
the name Kiwis give to thongs.*

Medical Nemesis

John Mukky Burke

We're happy, right? The doctors have waited.
Patients are strong for the new and shiny and not some piddly clinic
like in Ngukurr, Arakoon, not to mention Boree Creek.
Bring us your halt,
your lame, your weak, if you survive why not celebrate down the club?
There's heaps in Wagga.

Have I mentioned the RSL?

Funny Fog

Jean Burke

If words escape you,
                get lost on the journey

from brain to tongue,
from mind to sound,
just wait for them
to detour by
the tip
of your tongue,
somewhat apologetic,
late and relieved.

If words escape you,
                become lost completely,

waylaid in the deep woods,
just describe
their identifying features
as best you can:
paw nails for cats' claws
floor blanket for carpet,
which needs mowing,
a museum for water animals.

If words escape you,
                trans-form
in the haze of brain-fog
with a slip of the tongue,
just laugh
at the tricks your mind plays:
migraine into microwave,

elephant into envelope,
tourism into terrorism,
fog into funny.

making observations while under observation
Rosie Bogumil

a box of grey shutters the sky away
on this site of healing saturated by screaming
where requests are only ever denied.
for eggs.
for a smoke.
for some *fresh fucking air.*
even the orange paint seethes with rage:
what a strange colour for containment.
like our anger, good behaviour is here
rewarded in the worst ways.

the jam is always blackberry, squeezed
onto endless slices of bread with nothing
to spread it, nothing
to endanger ourselves
or others, us dangers to self.
every puzzle craves those few final pieces
while the winner of infinite rounds of cards
gambles chaos. much like the players,
the deck is mostly mismatched jokers.

our laughter is ingenuine,
manic. a finger pressed against warm lips warns:
be careful of that loose tongue of yours.
but whispers still collect between the sheets
within the walls, against the authoritarian fishbowl
and in the lens of security cameras perched in corners.
so many eyes are listening.
foreheads tickle from third-eye flutters but
we keep that sixth sense silent.

friendship is contraband. shoelaces though,
headphones and staples and
earrings and cables and
secrets inside an unsearched purse –
such a pity they could never match
the craftiness that comes with the crazy.

> 'need I remind you
> that your fellow patients
> are not your friends?
> relationships are frowned upon here.'

but I knew the girl who hung herself in room one.
we shared cigarettes beside
the no smoking sign.
they say she had *so much to live for*
and her rapist thought the same. *such* a pity.

even now, her room remains empty. haunted
I bought drugs from the boy in seven
before soaking the floor
of room four in blood, hoping
to drain away the darkness. later that night,
I used it for fingerpainting
but by the morning
the walls had been scrubbed clean.

The Z–A of Crazy
Alise Blayney

Zonk the over-zealous zeal of your zany zoomorphic zoom

You're yanked in Yonkers, *YES!*
You get the yolk for yakking down a Fat Yak while
yodelling a yummy yellow YALP and yelling
Yada yada yada.

Xylophones x-ray and revolt against the powers who believe they be —

With a wrought-up and wrong-headed wriggle, a wrathful worried worn.
Waxy rigidity has you whirlingly worked-up, wooden-headed with wondrous wit,
which you withered into witless woe.
Who's wary now, Witchypoo?
Wired, windy and wild with Warrior programming,
wigged out, whimsy and whacky wet!
Whisper your witzelsucht slapstick, non sequitur humour and wahneinfall wishes to a
Wendigo psychosis cannibal on skid row with walking corpse syndrome.
Want a well-built, well-lit wiretapped whacko who's weirded-out, weary, weak-minded and wayward?

Who's way-out wasteful, weaponised and warped with word salad and Wellbutrin wafers that wane and whisper to the whacko you are!

Voracious villains whose visions can be villainous and violent, and your vicious vile vibrates when very upset / very stupid / very lucid or very mad / bad and sad.
Varicoloured vapours vanish into voyeuristic vain and vague vacuous vacancy,
V2K: voice to skull technology.

Useless urgency makes you uptight, upside down, upset, upchucking upscale uproars upbeat, unzipped, and you're unthinkably untamed, unstrung and unsymmetrical.
Unspeakable things when unstrung, unsteady, unstable, unsound and unscrewed.
Unrestrained makes you unreasonable, unreal and unpredictable...
Unhinged and ungovernable when you've come undone.
Unleashing uncontrollable rifts of rage in Ursula's cave —
Usurping everyone!

Troubled mind is two-toned, two-fisted and twists Tourette's into turbulent tardive dyskinesia and targeted individual's synthetic telepathic torture at tribunal hearings to toke on trippy trivial tobacco addiction.
Traumatisation in vitro and counter transference
TREATMENT RESISTANT tortuous thunder!

Smiling surprisingly supernatural, superbly superhuman, suspicious when surreal, like suicidal strung-out strangers who suck the spirit out of spazzed-up spendthrifts, solicitous slant-wise splitting sociopaths, sinister sickos and shameless, seething senile, screwball schmucks who scrimp scandalous through this scamdemic, and spit savage with satanic ritual abuse panic!

Rage is raucous risk and runs ravage 'round the twist, rowdy and roughened, riotous and rattle-brained on a rapid eye movement rambling radical rampage!

Quease is questionable, quixotic and quirky with quantish

Puzzles of paranoid psychosis pumped puerile, predictive programming PSYOP projects provoking preposterous personality disordered pranks in poverty places of potty-mouthed possession of pockmark, poppycock perfectionist piles of pigshit phobic poison, pulsed with psionic inundation.
Plague plandemic and phrenetic phantoms in a psychogenic fugue of pyromaniac perversion with pea-brained police state, panic-strickened persnickety
Princess programmed Miss Piggy's!
PSYOP, PSYOP, with your pokey Project Paperclip prick: and I said hey, hey, Saint Peter, even your pointy phalanges look like the portal for PSYOP propaganda!

Over-worked into outlandish oppositional defiant, off-kilter Oedipal drama, obsessive compulsive Othello jealousy obliteration... Orchestrated Orwellian Order Ab Chao.
Oppressive Order out of Chao!

Nuisance nut-jobs with not the full shilling upstairs, not okay, not all there narcoleptic nightmares of non-symmetric neurolinguistic programming nonsense.
NON COMPOS MENTIS newfangledness.
Nauseatingly naïve and mysterious! Naïve on Neptune with the New World Order, naked with NASA (Never A Straight Answer).

Machiavellian multi-coloured mutton-headed mutations of motley moon-struck misfits,
Molotov cocktails mind-bogglingly messed up from the Mandela effect,
mentally deranged medleys of maniacal maladjusted,
MK-ULTRA and Monarch butterfly mind control with
MI5 lookin' mean on the MI6!

Mad-As-Hatter maniacs!

LIT LUNATIC, LIT LUNATIC, LIT LUNATIC!
LUNATICS, LET'S GET LIT!

Keyed-up kleptomaniacs stuck in a K-hole, keen on kaleidoscopic kuru and Korsakoff's syndrome to
KO the knight's move thinking, kangaroo court knuckleheaded killuminati
KAKISTOCRACY!

Jung's catalytic exteriorisation phenomenon jumps
Jackass jerky jackhammer juveniles

Irritated and irrational whilst intoxicated and irate —
insanely inhumane and inflamed.
Illusion des sosies — I think your pet Iguana is an imposter!
Inexplicably inconsiderate whilst incoherent —
idiosyncratic, impulsive and in-a-fit.

Hysterical hypochondria, huffy and high-strung, hot-headed and held-up. Hyde your Jekyll.
Hanging horrendously hospitalised — head over heels halting harebrained hallucinations...
Haste, you better run away then, and
Hyde your Jekyll!

Gung-ho and grotesque, grandiose and goosey, gang stalking Gestalt therapy
gonna go crazy, gone doolally, garish gander.
Grimoires and Goetia girls, grooming garbage in the Gulag

Fuming fuddled fury, fried-feeding frenzy,
frunk as duck and frantically foaming at the mouth,
fool hardily AND
frothing at the bit.
Four out of five voices in your head say go for it!
Flip your bush, flip your lid and wig, flip the fiendish fast times of

Excessive esoteric erotomaniac extremists, enraged and enraptured

Electra complex enthusiasts,

ECT candidates eliciting the embittered eccentric dunderhead who's

Dunce-like and dumpish, dull-witted Dhat syndrome dementia

dereistic thinking derailment déjà pensé

drooling dreadful dubious déjà vu drivel like me and my dehumanised

double-talk droogs who are dopey and doomed, dizzy, ditsy and

DISS MY PSYCHIATRIC DISABILITY like distorted, disgruntled ding-a-lings with

demonic delirium (tremendous tremens) and

debase dark triad traits with DSM-6 depressive dual diagnosis on a DSP, dissociated abilities with dark force entities!

Creeping on criminal crusades, cross-patched corrupt corkscrew coo-coos with

contorted clairvoyant convulsions,

controlling the weather by

CERN which/who/witch is a

CON-CERN,

Creating clouds of clairsentient consciousness and circumstantial speech with confabulated

clang associations that cut covert

Cheka counterintelligence into Claparede's paradox and disappear into Cotard delusions on

Community Treatment Orders!

Certifiable candidates for cray-cray covert narcissistic rage in

Bedlam's buffoonish broke-house for the brain sick, blindly boisterous bone heads, god blimey bizarro to

the big-ticketed bemused bats in the

BELFRY!

Beg your pardon about my Bipolar Bear who is backed by the

Burdekin Report, the

Burdekin Report!

Benevolently breaking barriers, barking brave and brazen,

bombastic breakthroughs with balls and backbone!

Applaud avant-garde acrimonious auto-maniacs, as keen as mustard and ardently aroused

alcohol use disordered Type A absurdists,

anarchistic altered

ADDICTS with akataphasia.

Alphabet agencies like ASIO anterograde amnesia and auditory agnosia with

acquired aphasia and

astasia-abasia of the

Alise in Wonderland experience fantasia!

Date Night

Sophie Bellotti

You look like a prisoner of war
as they march you up to the glass,
in your socks and the sweater I brought you
last time, which I thought would fit. Me,
with fresh makeup on since
school, itching under my coat in the
imposed comfort of the corridors.
Buttons pressed, doors
swung open, boundaries permeated. Later,
a monochromatic man offers us each a square
of iced vanilla cake, the type
that comes boxed, in a flimsy tinfoil tray.
We watch it sit there, perched
on a cardboard loveseat,
greenish. We won't touch it.
I'll stand and press my hand against
your fishbowl, tap incessantly on the glass.
My love not big enough;
Your love not big enough.
Until visiting hours
end at 8pm.

The Countdown

Ethan Bell

I know it ain't supposed to be. But I hurt the ones who get close to me

I ask that you pity not this deflated soul.
For when this lonely world has taken its toll

I will return to a starlight that shines bright in the night sky
Or maybe a madman shilling my own luxuries to all passers-by

I shall return to orange brown and grey like a cold winter's day
Or to a summer breeze, cooling a flushed red cheek

I account, that beauty surrounds me with each aching breath
Yet when I embrace the morning sun
All that I am, is awaiting death

I must confess another sin,
I fear my friends are blowing in the wind,

As the tree sap dries I hold on to the lies
The fear the anger the hurt the pain

I remained trapped in my broken heart
And fear that forever, I will remain, the same

I'm So Lonely

The Bedroom Philosopher

I'm so lonely
I spend my time playing Uno by myself
I'm so lonely
I only drink gin with Solo
The original mood crusher
On the stereo is One by U2
Followed by The Smashing Pumpkins
With Zero
I'm so lonely
My shadow wants to start seeing other people
I'm so lonely
I top and tail with myself in a single bed
A euphemism for the foetal position
I spend my time reading through my old diaries
I can only live through myself vicariously
I'm getting intensely jealous of my own memories
All my imaginary friends used to be real
I'm the thirteenth sign of the zodiac
It is a hole that is black
The goldfish remembers to turn its back
I ran a bubble bath it went flat
I had a falling out
I'm not talking to myself anymore

Sestina: Rape

Stuart Barnes

i.m. Anita Cobby

When I was a kid it hid in our red crêpe
paper crowns, the scrape
of fair knees, my mother's grape
hyacinths. At eight I watched it fly from behind a drape,
the nation-shocking abduction, gang-rape
and murder of Anita Cobby. Nirvana's 'Rape

Me', Tori Amos' 'Me And A Gun'—white grape
-fruit. I was eighteen when DATE-RAPE
donged. *'No such thing as male rape'*
flared. No rape report, no rape
kit. When I split the pith of this rape
three sweethearts laughed in my face. Rape

bird-dogged me—the grapevine, the sky-scrape
-red air; crepe myrtle, broomrape;
crêpes Suzette, red grape
-fruit. I squirmed at university—Zeus' rape
of Leda, her nape caught in his bill; trape
-zius myalgia fanning out; the scrape

of pear trees. Rape
-enclosure, my fourth sweetheart. Hard rape
counselling. I forced down *Law & Order: SVU*—rape
-exposure after rape
-exposure—finally, I stopped the keen. Rape
-opiates? All stepped down. I cared for myself with rape

(*Brassica napus*). I devoured rape.
I cleaned my teeth with the bones of rape.
I was forty when GANG-RAPE

gonged. I was mellow as rape
vinegar. I pared terror like grape
-fruit. Two beloveds denied my rape

-song. Seven repaired my red trape
-ze. It opened me like a window, this rape.
Here, see its material drape:

```
   r            a p              e
   r           a    p            e
   r         a        p          e
   r       a            p        e
   r     a                p      e
   r   a                    p    e
   r     a                 p     e
   r       a             p       e
   r         a         p         e
```

Rape declared nuclear war, but I am not rape
-torn or -weary, a rape trophy or poet. Rape,
I've got my eye on you. Rape, prepare. ~~Rape.~~

Inertia

Spencer Barberis

A widowed fluorescent shudders bleach over malignant linoleum
in a kitchen
      with not enough bench space.

A too steep spiral staircase ascends to the second floor
of a house
      soon to be demolished.

Water stains bloom across the ceiling like
           memories eroding holes in whites and greys
above rooms coated autumnal
by afternoons filtered
through fading
bedsheet curtains.

None of us were on the lease.

We were the seventh season of that house
maybe the eighth
and the writers were getting sloppy.
Communal box wine. Communal chop bowl.
Communal pube trimming scissors
          bleeding outlines in the shower.

I was quick switching between states
the way heat applied to a solid
can make a liquid
can make a vapour.
      Sweet like a kiss.
      Nice like it wants something.

There were things I didn't know that I knew.

       weeks / when I / could barely / speak / but made / a chorus /
       with / the white goods / my body / atrophied / by thought /
(then)
       legs like pistons everything about me in flight endless ideas
       crippled by their size my mouth and eyes talking everyone
       into bed and a rage this fucking rage opaque like burnt glass
       myself and my anger holding each other down

She yelled at me
              Be better
              Just be better
And I wanted to be better.
I did.
     I really did.

                       But actually I didn't.
What I wanted was complete combustion
      though I could hardly move
      for the things
         I had done.

I drove too fast on midnight arteries through red lights in a car that
would soon be scrapped with a friend I would soon fall out with.
They were trying to talk me down but my arguments were too
compelling and too shrill. At The Gap I thought about my mother and
the blood that would be on my hands and how I didn't want to die,
not really, just wanted

            immersion
      in a darkness removed from dichotomy
         without noise but not silence
          just something outside of it
    not awake and not asleep and not dreaming either
           just something other
             than any of this
         I wanted to be suspended

static
in air moving so fast it becomes viscous
so swift I become a stillness

but a fall from that height
or any really
would have just been too short
for that.

The Key

Mary Baker

As free as a bird in a cage,
You have trapped me.
And thrown away the key.

The key to my happiness,
To my life. So that I am flying in circles,
Going nowhere. Achieving nothing.

You have taken over,
Like the co-pilot of a plane,
When the captain loses control.

But I hadn't lost it.
I knew what I was doing;
I know what I am doing.

Maybe it will be different this time,
Maybe I can change.
You cannot know unless you try.

So unravel this cocoon of your protection,
Untie this chain of your love.
Open the door, release me.

Trust that I won't fly away.
But if I do,
Trust that it is for the best.

Let go of the past.
Let go of your fear.
Let go of my hand.

Free us both.
From each other.
You have the key.

Reflections on 'The Key'

Annette and Stuart Baker

I aim to promote awareness and acceptance of these illnesses which are so often ignored. With knowledge and understanding, we can come out of the shadows and move forwards to a brighter future.
Mary Baker

Annette and Stu Baker lost their daughter Mary to suicide at age fifteen. Alongside her passions for horseriding and water polo, Mary found a real love for poetry through her English class at school.

Annette

I see myself in the poem as the primary holder of the key and for this, I carry an enduring sadness.

That Mary was unable ever, even in the depths of her illness, to reveal her pain and suffering leaves me as her mother with deep regret and sorrow.

In this, I believe she was protecting us from the knowledge that one day she would fly away.

Mary's major school English project *Out of the Shadows* opened her eyes to what was possible for her to say in poetry that she couldn't and wasn't able to physically convey with words.

I consider her poetry and prose about mental health as a gift and it has been the catalyst for our activism. Some have said she's left a legacy.

Stuart

I first read Mary's poem 'The Key' three days after her death.

My overwhelming feelings were sadness, understanding, and gratitude.

Mary has expressed the anguish and pain of her mental ill-health and the role she and we played in the three years of battling an eating disorder in our quest to return to normal.

The poem doesn't offer hope of recovery and the sadness for me is in understanding that our ultimately failed attempt to return Mary to full health inflicted a very heavy toll on her emotional wellbeing.

The key is used metaphorically throughout the poem both to denote our control of Mary's freedom and the hold her illness has over her.

The repetition of the theme of being trapped and confined in the early stanzas of the poem builds an image of despair at the illness and the familial control.

In the final stanzas the poem talks of freedom, release, and trust in the unknown as if to offer an answer.

* In the days following Mary's death and in the depths of our grief we wrote to the two surviving poets whose poems Mary analysed.

The first response was from Les Murray who had suffered from depression and his letter has been a comfort to us.

His first sentence read: 'What a filthy unjust thing mental illness can be, taking away a life that clearly had every reason to be happy and proud of itself'.

Episode(s)

Mohammad Awad

A therapist's voice
grating,

Search for cracks of light
in empty corners,
Rest your head where Devil's Ivy
could not survive,
Feel its earth for nourishment,
Notice its desert texture,
Notice how neither of you have been watered
in weeks,

Breathe in,
        Count the amount of times
        your father ever held you
        in positive regard,
Breathe out.

Don't look at your reflection.

You may see an intruder in your body,
        An abuser in your body,
        A stranger—

Protruding frame,
Hips you can't body shame away,
Swallowing your gut as you end this verse,

You may see failed attempts
        at living
            and dying,

I hope you find success in some part of life.

Search for euphoria
at the depths of dysphoria,
Find contentment
in the climax of all tension,
Grip *firmly* onto sharp objects,
Avoid regrettable intentions,
Each thought a dagger,
Slicing, Shaping, Carving

My World
is half what it was this morning,
A fraction of what it was yesterday,
There is no knowing
what the next hour will bring.

My morning begins
in most people's afternoons,

I am no night owl insomniac,
I am sunrise that sets   in the south.

I am the moon—   split
and spat upon,
Orbiting incorrect planets
in distant solar systems,
Black sheep
in nuclear human family.

Therapist speaks
to me as I—
Clutch to carpet,

Still trying to convince me
To find cracks of light,

I am still trying to convince
My lungs,
Oxygen has not left the room.

Interior Anxious

Evelyn Araluen

My interior scrapes
furniture across a floor I won't clean
dressing windows with dreams
that don't look me in the eye

Nothing's quiet at night
when you make it your only living
light breaks   so much
and ghosts aren't meant for the day

My insides sleep in doorways
        like I'm waiting for this to fall
outside the wattle bird cracks dusk from dawn
where the moon slips blue eyed
through the slivers I allow myself
to give her glimpse of how far it's gone

I know every crevice of this crypt
its soft   its sorry   its sleeping
but this house is not home, is not a hearth to tend
or a corner to curl in curtain glow
I promised you I'd clear space in this aching mess
but you've never seen   such a clutter rupture
        never held such an empty pen

I'm tearing shadows from the dark
teaching myself to dream in repetition
            spirit and spectre dance silhouettes through halls
            while I watch seasick and desert-mouthed this
            fluorescent holocene screen tracing
            room to hollow room

dangling feet from every edge

to test how much living wants

    I don't want to call   just to
write in white to give the empty something to eat
without showing the bones:
        they said what you give space will be given
        before time
        in a future past this present
            split-ribboned by what we refused
            what wasn't ours to keep
but we don't get time every way that we want it
and we don't get what we want every time
you told me: give it a morning to unpack and a night to breathe out
        if it crawls out the window
        it was never meant to be housed

None of this is to say that I'm healing
        or that what's here is ready to rest
it says   I lost my days to my mind
I didn't get what I wanted
when I gave it my time
now my interior hoards light like I don't deserve it
playing dressup in disasters that wear like paper dolls

It's to say   we're grasping through distance and disorder
and I'm still here, despite a history conspiring to kill me
        but the unutterable of living
        when you make living a choice
        is that a mind can make monotony of anything
        can drag bodies room to room
        till the horror
        is a floating sheet
        in a dusty house

From the window
             this looks like breaking
from the sky
it's only ghost

Better Out Than In

Christine Anu

I feel gagged sometimes censored of the words I wish to speak
So I close my eyes and in the darkness I'm on a mountain peak

From way up high the words I cry of my true misery
My one safe place is where I know I am sheltered, I am free

It is a nightmare, it is a dream, what is real I cannot know I
do know, when I do wake, is what I reap from what I sow

The thing that's real is when I open my eyes, the mask I choose to wear
To stand before a sea of faces with judging eyes that stare

Milky haze, meet silky days
The confusion makes me want to shout
So I close my eyes, to the mountain top I go and scream,

'Just let me out!'

Sexual Assault Report Questionnaire: Describe your hair.

Eunice Andrada

What would happen if one woman told the truth about her life? The
world would split open.
Muriel Rukeyser, 'Käthe Kollwitz'

Of the sixteen kinds of breakage, often it chooses
to crack into right angles. What this says about me:
I coil my crown into unforgiving shapes.
The categories of damage creeping up my hair:
basic splits, baby splits, deep splits, long splits,
triple splits, double y splits, like a roll call

for failed efforts of resistance. The counsellor calls
for our regular phone sessions, asks me to choose
what I want to talk about. I reach up to my uncombable hair:
knots, trees, candles, feathers, offshoots, incomplete splits.
The reminders come. I'm told to notice what's around me.
Tally the yellow objects in the room. Note the pattern of shapes.

In the recurring math problem, it asks which shape
of vessel can hold the heaviest shame. I call
a friend—white spots, thickened ends, crinkle splits,
right angles—*why did you have to come to me?*
The beeping admits a worthier emergency. I must choose
for myself. I wring the answer from my hair.

On average, women spend 1.5 years doing their hair
with their unique combination of scorched shape
-shifting, chemical colouring—Vivian compliments me
on my buzzed head outside the library. I choose
not to submit the report. What will they call
a girl not the right colour or demeanour, no split

hem? I tell the truth and expect the world to split
open. Fissures crawl up the length of my hair
to prove its tolerance. When I was younger, I'd choose
to spend summers chewing on my ponytail. They'd call
me away from my gnawing, not knowing what shaped
the daydreams: my lineage or me.

When I watch robins plummet from the sky, it's just me.
A poet asks, what feminine part of yourself did you split
off clean so you wouldn't be catcalled?
Even in garish light I can't recognise the shapes
behind car windows. The growth cycle of hair
on your scalp is 2 to 7 years. You can't choose.

Nachos

Steph Amir

i.   *A few questions*
Are you sure you locked the door? Is that blood there on the
floor? Why's that person looking pale? How many hands have
touched my mail? I wonder why my friend just frowned. Does
she not want me around? Do I *have to* eat that pie? Should
have I just told them why I had to leave that crowded place?
Or couldn't kiss my daughter's face? How long's *too* long to
wash my hands? How many handshakes can I stand? Should I
stay here at my desk, trapped in scenes of gore and sex? Should
I try to walk it off? Could I *ever* tell my boss? Why suddenly
do I feel dizzy? Is it that I'm just too busy? Hormones? Am I
stressed, or sick? Do I need to get out quick? What if I faint,
puke or scream? What if that doorknob's not clean? Why *am* I
seeing blood again? Am I officially *insane*?

ii.   *The Yale-Brown Obsessive Compulsive Scale*
Fear of cheating? Insect spray?
Washing many times a day?
Avoiding throwing things away?
Worrying, "What if I'm gay?"

Checking locks without delay?
Sticky substance: honey? Clay?
Thoughts that never go away:
Cancer? Black cats? Knives, you say...?

iii.   *The principles of transcranial magnetic stimulation for OCD*
Heterogeneity of neuroanatomy –
OCD is in the community:

Dysregulation of cortical activity,
Behaviours to reduce anxiety,
Broad mix of obsessions and severity.

Magnets induce neural electricity,
Titrated from the minimum intensity.
Precise modulation of cortical activity
Increases useful connectivity,
With the possibility of metaplasticity.

iv. *Today*

I dream about how one day, I'll reach out and open the door of
a restaurant; a friend's house; any door. I'll travel anywhere,
even places where the guidebooks say the water's not safe to
drink. I'll stop planning for illnesses that never happen; realise
it's been a while since I was last blinded by violent fictions.

But not today.

Today I wash my hands, double-check the locks, and walk
down the street avoiding suspicious stains. I sit down with
my friends, ignore the battle of self-versus-self, focus on my
newly-reinforced neural circuits, and before I can change
my mind, I start eating nachos, not with my usual socially-
awkward fork from a snap-lock bag but WITH MY OWN BARE
FINGERS and it's just as delicious as I hoped it would be.

Notes

Text in part ii is taken from the Yale-Brown Obsessive Compulsive Scale, the
most commonly used tool to diagnose obsessive compulsive disorder.

Except for the word 'clay', text in part iii is taken from: Luca Cocchi, Andrew
Zalesky, Zoie Nott, Geneviève Whybird, Paul B. Fitzgerald and Michael
Breakspear, 'Transcranial magnetic stimulation in obsessive-compulsive
disorder: a focus on network mechanisms and state dependence', *NeuroImage:
Clinical*, 2018, vol. 19, pp. 661–674.

Toilet Stall Poetry

Maja Amanita

They took the hook off the back of the toilet doors at the psychiatric hospital,
And I'm wondering if the lady in the next stall is crying for the same reason

annexiety

Claire Albrecht

anxiety is the millennial condition, says a click-bait article I
probably read somewhere; as for my own tangles, well,
there are some parties you just shouldn't go to.
I'm one gnarled shoot of a gnarly nervous system,

jacked up on caffeine-free cokes and celery and
clenching my teeth at that cunt of a waiter, who probably
had a panic attack five minutes ago. this basically
makes us sisters. 'you aren't lazy, you're just terrified'

is the latest feel-good production of the meme machine, but
I can tell you right now, I'm definitively both – don't pretend
they're mutually exclusive. I can drop a potato chip
down the sleeve of my knitted jumper while I fear for

all our futures, eye the vacuum off for months feeling petrified
of filling one. but what's a bit of dust floating around? at night
I try to dream of Putin, just to see what he'd be like,
shirtless, playing piano, I'm sprawled naked on his lounge

stringing cheese between my fingers and feeling the soft-
ness of what's probably bear pelt tucked up under my arse.
I tell him he can sanction and annex whatever he likes,
if he promises not to meddle with my domestic affairs and

we watch porn together, tapes of Trump pissing on women,
he tells me his fantasies and I tell him mine, and when I try
to fuck him from behind he gets antsy, grunts out a veto,
something about NATO and the security of his borders and

I get bored again, make a smoothie and sit cross-legged on
my deck watching bats. things like, do you think Princess Diana
liked pineapple on her pizza? not a metaphor, but I'd be interested
either way. my earrings shake in the air like icicles in an earthquake.

Notes

'Frequency', Jenny Hedley

1   'Memories sometimes come backwards. They haunt-walk in.' Ellen van Neerven, *Throat*

2   'Guilt says, I made a mistake. Shame says, I am a mistake.' Lucia Osborne-Crowley, *I Choose Elena*

3   'The longer a physical assault or accident is held in the nervous system, the muscles and the brain, without being addressed or treated, the more likely it is that it will manifest as a systemic physical disorder or dysfunction.' Osborne-Crowley

IF I SMELL GAS AND THERE IS NO GAS or AM I A PSYCHOANALYST IF I DON'T HAVE A COUCH? Pascalle Burton

1   Aase Berg, 'Language and Madness' (translated by Johannes Göransson and Joyelle McSweeney), *Poetry Foundation*, 3 April 2019, https://tinyurl.com/22bvpt5x.

2   'The evolution of the psychoanalyst's office', *CBS News*, 19 May 2013, https://tinyurl.com/2s3vxp8b.

3   Daniel Zola, 'Reclaiming personhood against the rise of mental health discourse', *Overland*, 14 October 2021, https://tinyurl.com/3t7rayja.

4   Nathan Filer, *The Heartland: Finding and Losing Schizophrenia*, London: Faber and Faber, 2019, p. 195.

5   EM Greenhalgh, S Jenkins, S Stillman & C Ford, '7.12 Smoking and mental health', in *Tobacco in Australia: Facts and Issues*, eds E Greenhalgh, M Scollo & M Winstanley, Melbourne: Cancer Council Victoria, 2018, https://tinyurl.com/2p8wm2dj.

6   Filer, *The Heartland*, pp. 120–121.

7   Jane Dykema, 'What I Don't Tell My Students About "The Husband Stitch"', *Electric Literature*, 10 October 2017, https://tinyurl.com/4k34t6s2.

8   Filer, *The Heartland*, p. 172.

9   Tobias Carrol, '"I had zero allegiance to realism": an interview with Lidia Yuknavitch', *Vol. 1 Brooklyn*, 20 July 2015, https://tinyurl.com/2p969s79.

10   Lidia Yuknavitch's Twitter account, 12 January 2022, https://tinyurl.com/3m3ay9dr.

11   Jon Caramanica, 'The peerless imagination of Greg Tate', *The New York Times*, 8 December 2021, https://tinyurl.com/2p8j7jbd.

12   Greg Tate, *Flyboy 2: The Greg Tate Reader*,Durham, NC: Duke University Press, 2016, p. 9.

13   James Hannaham, *Pilot Imposter*, New York: Soft Skull Press, 2021, p. 1.

14   Gold cited in Filer, *The Heartland*, p. 178.

15   bell hooks, *All about Love: New Visions*, New York: HarperCollins, 2000, pp. 5, 101.

Sestina: Rape, Stuart Barnes

The phrase 'her nape caught in his bill' is from W. B. Yeats' 'Leda and the Swan'.

Nachos, Steph Amir

Text from part ii taken from the *Yale-Brown Obsessive Compulsive Scale*, the most commonly used tool to diagnose obsessive compulsive disorder.

Text from part iii including the subtitle is taken from an academic paper by Australian neurology and psychiatry researchers: Luca Cocchi, Andrew Zalesky, Zoie Nott, Geneviève Whybird, Paul B. Fitzgerald and Michael Breakspear, 'Transcranial magnetic stimulation in obsessive-compulsive disorder: a focus on network mechanisms and state dependence', *NeuroImage: Clinical*, 2018, vol. 19, pp. 661–674.

Words from both texts have been reordered so the original meaning is not necessarily retained. Edits to individual words are indicated with brackets. The grammar is the poet's own.

Contributors

Manal Younus is a storyteller who believes that language and stories are the very fabric of our existence. Originally from Eritrea and raised on Kaurna Country in South Australia, she uses her writing and performance to create experiences that encourage audiences to join her in asking questions of themselves and the world around them. In 2015 she released her first book of poetry, called *Reap*, and launched it with a national tour. She has since gone on to perform at schools and events around the country and the world, including at the Jaipur Literary Festival and George Town Literary Festival.

Fiona Wright is a writer, editor and critic. Her book of essays *Small Acts of Disappearance* won the 2016 Kibble Award and the Queensland Literary Award and was shortlisted for the 2016 Stella Prize. Her poetry collections are *Knuckled* and *Domestic Interior*, and her new essay collection is *The World Was Whole*.

Jennifer Wong is a Chinese Australian writer, comedian, and food enthusiast from Sydney. She writes about food, culture and mental health, and has been published by ABC Everyday, SBS Food, and *Monocle*. As a comedian, she's performed in arts and comedy festivals in Australia, Edinburgh and Shanghai. As a food enthusiast, she's the presenter of *Chopsticks or Fork?*, a six-part ABC series about Chinese restaurants in regional Australia. Jennifer's experience with depression began in 2002. A hospital stay in 2018 led to the writing of the viral article 'Ten things I'm slowly learning about recovery from depression' for ABC Everyday.

Misbah Wolf writes prose poetry and short stories. Her work has had the good fortune of being accepted through many great journals – *APJ*, *Mascara Literary Journal*, *Peril*, *Cordite*, and upcoming work in *Overland*, and in anthologies like *Solid Air* and *Contemporary*

Asian Australian Poets. Following on from her acclaimed first book, *Rooftops in Karachi*, is her second book, *Carapace*, ,coming out in May 2022 through Vagabond Press, which explores mental illness, drugs, sex and relationships formed in the cicada-like shell of share-housing.

Arlea Whelan is twenty-one and studies creative writing at the University of Wollongong. She loves spoken word poetry, karate, post-it notes and following Jesus. Much of her writing is about painful experiences, but she thinks any poem can be beautiful if it hits the soul at the right angle.

Wart is an artist and has over forty years of experience exhibiting and performing. Wart also lives with a Mental Illness and has been an advocate and worker in this field in the Arts. Her last exhibition was funded by a Create NSW Grant primarily and a City of Sydney one for the weekend talks. The show was called EYE SEE PINK BLACK AND WHITE. It looked at scrutiny and beauty and ideas of stigmatisation. Wart's work is humorous, deep, socially evocative and thought provoking. Wart's wordwork and paintings have been collected in her recent book *Past Wents*, published by Apothecary Archive.

Grown from a carob pod in a sunny, Central Coast national park, **Felicity Ward** is a multi-award-winning comedian, actor and writer who has performed across Australia, North America and the UK. A hilarious, undeniable force of energy on stage, she has been nominated for Most Outstanding Show at both the Melbourne International Comedy Festival and the Edinburgh Fringe, with her live comedy specials featuring on Netflix and the BBC. She has appeared on TV screens in Australia and abroad, from *Spicks and Specks* to the UK's *Live at the Apollo* and *Mock the Week*, as well as a dramatic turn in ABC TV's *Wakefield*. As an advocate for mental health awareness, she also hosted the ABC documentary *Felicity Ward's Mental Mission* and regularly speaks at mental health charities and organisations.

Susie Walsh is a poet, writer, and filmmaker. Her poem 'Discordant' was in the Solastalgia exhibition (Tuggeranong Arts Centre, 2020) and her poem 'How I Hold You' is in *What We Carry* (Recent Works Press,

2021). Susie is working on *Palimpsest*, her first collection of poems and hybrid texts.

Ellen van Neerven is a Mununjali writer and editor. They are the author of three books: *Heat and Light* (UQP, 2014), *Comfort Food* (UQP, 2016), and *Throat* (UQP, 2020).

Sam Twyford-Moore is the author of *The Rapids: Ways of Looking at Mania*, which was published by NewSouth Publishing in 2018 and the University of Toronto Press in 2020. His new book, *Cast Mates*, a popular history of Australian actors working in America, is forthcoming from NewSouth.

Lindsay Tuggle is the author of *The Afterlives of Specimens*, which was glowingly reviewed in *The New York Review of Books*. Her debut poetry collection, *Calenture*, was named one of *The Australian's* Books of the Year, shortlisted for the Association for the Study of Australian Literature's Mary Gilmore Award and the Australian Poetry Foundation's Anne Elder Award. Lindsay won the prestigious Kluge Fellowship at the Library of Congress, alongside fellowships from the Mütter Museum and the Australian Academy of the Humanities. She is concurrently writing a second poetry collection, *The Autopsy Elegies*, and a work of biological fiction, *The Whisper Sisters*.

Elizabeth Tan is the author of *Rubik* (2017), a novel-in-stories, and *Smart Ovens for Lonely People* (2020), a collection of short stories which won the 2020 Readings Prize for New Australian Fiction. Her recent writing has appeared in *Portside Review*, *Dear Mum*, *Liminal* and *Silent Dialogue*. She lives in Boorloo/Perth.

Cher Tan is an essayist and critic in Naarm/Melbourne, via Kaurna Yerta / Adelaide and Singapore. Her work has appeared in the *Sydney Review of Books*, *Runway Journal*, *Overland*, *The Lifted Brow*, *Kill Your Darlings* and *Gusher* magazine, among others. She is the reviews editor at *Meanjin* and an editor at *Liminal*.

Grace Tame is an outspoken advocate for survivors of sexual assault, particularly those who were abused in institutional settings. From age fifteen, Grace was groomed and raped by her 58-year-old maths teacher, who was found guilty and jailed for his crimes. However, under Tasmania's sexual-assault victim gag laws, Grace couldn't legally speak out about her experience – despite the perpetrator and media being free to do so. Grace has demonstrated extraordinary courage, using her voice to push for legal reform and raise public awareness about the impacts of sexual violence. In 2021 Grace was recognised as the Australian of the Year, the *Australian Financial Review*'s most culturally powerful person and one of *Time* magazine's next generation leaders.

David Stavanger is a poet, cultural producer, editor and former psychologist living on unceded Dharawal land. His first full-length poetry collection, *The Special* (UQP, 2014), was awarded the Arts Queensland Thomas Shapcott Poetry Prize and the Wesley Michel Wright Poetry Prize. David co-directed Queensland Poetry Festival (2015–2017). He is the co-editor of *Australian Poetry Journal* 8.2 – 'spoken', *Rabbit* 27 – Tense, and *Solid Air: Collected Australian & New Zealand Spoken Word* (UQP, 2019.) His latest collection, *Case Notes* (UWAP, 2020), won the 2021 Victorian Premier's Literary Award for Poetry.

Anna Spargo-Ryan is a Melbourne writer, the author of two novels and a winner of the Horne Prize. Her new book, *A Kind of Magic*, is a blended memoir about life – and joy – with serious mental illness.

Samson J. L. Soulsby is a queer writer, editor, and academic living on unceded Dharawal country. His fiction and poetry have featured in *Legacies Anthology* and *Baby Teeth Journal* and his writing is forever haunted by monsters, plants, magic, light, darkness, hope, rot, love, transformation and madness.

Brooke Scobie is a queer Goorie single mum, poet, writer, podcaster and community worker. Her writing is a love letter to people who've been systematically excluded. She's been published in *Overland*,

Running Dog, Red Room Poetry, SBS, *Best of Australian Poems 2021*, and was awarded second place in the 2020 Judith Wright Poetry Prize.

Kirli Saunders is a proud Gunai Woman and award-winning writer, artist, and consultant. An experienced speaker and facilitator advocating for the environment, gender, racial equality and LGBTIQA+ rights, Kirli was the NSW Aboriginal Woman of the Year (2020). In 2022, She received at OAM for her contribution to the arts and literature, her books include *The Incredible Freedom Machines* (Scholastic, 2018), *Kindred* (Magabala, 2019), *Bindi* (Magabala, 2020), *Our Dreaming* (Scholastic, 2022) and *Returning* (Magabala, 2023).

Sara M. Saleh is an award-winning poet, writer, human rights activist and the daughter of migrants from Palestine, Egypt and Lebanon, currently living on Gadigal land. Her pieces have been published in various national and international outlets and anthologies and her debut novel, *Songs for the Dead and the Living*, is out in 2023.

Omar Sakr is the author of *These Wild Houses* (Cordite, 2017) and *The Lost Arabs* (UQP, 2019), which won the 2020 Prime Minister's Literary Award for Poetry. His poems have been widely published and anthologised in places such as the Academy of American Poets Poem-a-Day series, *Border Lines: Poems of Migration* (Vintage Knopf, 2020), *Anthology of Australian Prose Poetry* (MUP, 2020), *Best Australian Poems* (Black Inc., 2016) and *Contemporary Australian Poetry* (Puncher & Wattmann, 2016). Born and raised on Dharug country to Lebanese and Turkish Muslim migrants, he lives there still. His debut novel, *Son of Sin* (2022), is out now with Affirm Press.

Rebecca Rushbrook is a mama, a photographer, an administrative assistant, an English tutor, a poetry editor, and a published and performance poet living in the Northern Rivers town of Lismore, New South Wales. She is a 2020 Australian Poetry Slam NSW finalist, a Nimbin Performance Poetry Cup winner, and three-times winner of the Lismore Poetry Cup. Rebecca edited the Newcastle Fringe Festival anthology, *poesis*. She has been published in the MTV Books Saul Williams anthology, *Chorus*, and the Sydney Writers' Festival anthology, *Litlink*. Her poem 'Mine' featured in the anti-CSG movie *Rock the Gate* and became a protest poem text for high school study.

Anne Rachael Ross is a poet and writer. She grew up in glen innes (Ngarbal country) and completed degrees in writing and literature and chemistry at the university of wollongong. She has work published on Red Room, *Baby Teeth Journal* and *#EnbyLife*. She is working on a novel and a collection of poetry. She is a Christian and a transgender woman.

Paris Rosemont is a poet with a passion for the arts. She has crafted award-winning poetry that has been described as visceral hyperrealism. Having received a scholarship to study at the *Australian Theatre for Young People*, Paris hopes to combine her love for poetry and theatre into the exploration of the art of performance poetry. Paris is currently a WestWords 2022 Academian and a Frontier Poetry scholarship recipient.

Lillian Rodrigues-Pang is a professional oral storyteller of Pipil and Palestinian descent living on Dharawal lands. She has been sharing the heart and power of story within Australian and international theatres and festival main-stages for over 20 years. When she is not on stage or creating cultural events she is sharing story love in the community as a connective, teaching and healing art. She is still living the lived experience.

Ariel Riveros Pavez is an award-winning writer who is based in Sydney. His poetry and prose work have appeared in various reviews and journals, nationally and internationally.

Tess Ridgway is a poet and comedian living on Gadigal land. She has a Master's of Research from Western Sydney University. Her poetry has been published in *Overland, Griffith Review* and *Otoliths*.

Michelle Rickerby has written film reviews in London and short-form content for children's television. Her poems have appeared in *Blume Illustrated, fourW* and two multi-artform exhibitions. She edited *In*

Case of Fire: An Anthology of Blue Mountains Poetry, (Spinebill Press, 2022). Michelle writes and edits in the Blue Mountains.

Bhenji Ra is a transdisciplinary artist based on Gadigal land, Eora Nation. Her practice combines dance, video, illustration and community activation. Her work dissects cultural theory and identity, centralising her own personal histories as a tool to reframe performance. She is the mother of Western Sydney-based collective and ballroom House of Slé.

Hope One is a Takatāpui Beatboxer, Writer, Performer, and Mother from Te Ātihaunui-a-Papārangi and Taranaki iwi of Aotearoa, fusing together Beatboxing, Spoken Word, Drag and Movement to deliver captivating Beat Rhyming experiences about identity, culture, queerness, motherhood and navigating trauma.

Steven Oliver is a writer/performer and is a descendant of the Kuku-Yalanji, Waanyi, Gangalidda, Woppaburra, Bundjalung and Biripi peoples. He was born in Cloncurry in North West Queensland and grew up in Townsville. His poetry is published in both national and international poetry journals such as *Ora Nui, Australian Poetry Journal, Solid Air* and *Firefront*. His plays *Proppa Solid* (Jute Theatre) and *From Darkness* (La Boite Theatre) are also published (Playlab). His one-man cabaret show *Bigger & Blacker* has toured nationally.

Comedian and mental health advocate **Nat's What I Reckon** rocketed into global prominence with his isolation cooking content. Nat has delivered a well-received talk for TEDx Sydney in which he examined the perception of success, was an ambassador for the Big Anxiety festival and has shared his coping technique ("taking the piss") on the Stand Up For Mental Health showcase for ABC TV. Nat's first and second books were awarded Booktopia's Favourite Australian Book Award with Nat donating the prize money to mental health charity Beyond Blue. Both books have been shortlisted in the prestigious Australian Book Industry Awards. With a message of inclusivity, positivity and never punching down, Nat's positive impact on the mental health of millions cannot be underestimated.

Anisa Nandaula is a nationally recognised spoken word poet, playwright, educator and published author. She is the 2016 Queensland Poetry slam champion. In 2017 she published her first book, *Melanin Garden*, and won Queensland Poetry Festival's XYZ Innovation in Spoken Word Prize. In 2018 she wrote, directed and starred in the play *The Grass is Dead on the Other Side* at the Brisbane Powerhouse. In 2019 she wrote and acted in the spoken word theatre show *How to Spell Love* that was showcased at the Judith Wright Centre. Anisa is also the co-founder of the arts collective Voices of Colour, which creates spaces for migrant, refugee and First Nations artists to share their work.

Lotovale Junior Nanai was – and always will be – a poet. Born in Falelatai, Western Samoa, in January 1982 (deceased 2022), Junior came to Australia when he was one. He lived in the Illawarra and first performed his poetry at the MAD Poetry event at the 2019 Wollongong Writers Festival. Junior loved life and concentrated on improvisation and phone text poetry. *Vale Junior, your MAD Poetry family misses your light.*

Omar Musa is a Bornean-Australian author, visual artist and poet from Queanbeyan, Australia. He has released four poetry books (including *Killernova*) and four hip-hop records, and received a standing ovation at TEDx Sydney at the Sydney Opera House. His debut novel, *Here Come the Dogs*, was longlisted for the International Dublin Literary Award and Miles Franklin Award, and he was named one of the *Sydney Morning Herald*'s Young Novelists of the Year in 2015. His one-man play, *Since Ali Died*, won Best Cabaret Show at the Sydney Theatre Awards in 2018. He has had several solo exhibitions of his woodcut prints.

Melanie Mununggurr is a Djapu woman, mother, poet, storyteller and performer. Her writing speaks on her identity as queer, First Nations and being mother to a child with special needs. Melanie uses her connection to her country and her language to decolonise the literary and performance space through the use of Dhuwal language weaved throughout her poems. Melanie has a book of poetry to be published in the near future by Penguin Random House and is working, writing, directing and performing in her first show, with world-renowned beatboxer Hope One.

Scott-Patrick Mitchell is a Boorloo-based non-binary poet. Their poem in this anthology discusses their thirty-plus years lived experience of travelling with suicidal ideation. They are also a reformed methamphetamine addict, which they have written about in their first full-length poetry collection, *Clean*, also available from Upswell Publishing.

Misha the maniac (aka Michael Alexandratos) is an alter-ego and nom de guerre that was created as an outlet to express and articulate in creative form the author's lived experiences with psychosis, anorexia and other mental health conditions. They live in Sydney and are working on various archival, research and publishing projects.

Avowing that nothing-other-than-poetry allows one to be so disallowed, **D.L. Marcus**'s practice grapples to express inexpressible limits of suffering. To narrate the disintegration of a previous self, language must fracture like kaleidoscopic episode. Yet Marcus maintains the inverse relationship here also holds true: that poetry can reassemble and seal fractured selves.

Anthony Mannix was born in 1953 in Sydney. Studying cultural anthropology at Macquarie University, he felt an avenue to explore reality and unreality in a continuous book of 'subjective documentation' of text and art. For the last thirty-six years he has pursued this. Anthony is widely exhibited and published. In 2019 he released his collected writings, *The Toy of the Spirit*, available through Puncher & Wattmann. More of Anthony's work and images of his original artist books can be found in his digital archive, *The Atomic Book*, at www.apothecaryarchive.com.

Gemma Mahadeo has been based on Wurundjeri land since 1987. They are a queer, non-binary poet and writer whose work has appeared in national and international journals online and in print. They are also a disability advocate, being one of the founding members of The Disabled QBIPOC Collective. They love and play lots of music, and sometimes review beer on eatdrinkstagger.com.

Chris Lynch is a white New Guinean-Australian of Gaelic ancestry who lives alongside the Merri Creek, on Wurundjeri Country. He is working on a novel.

Rozanna Lilley's work has appeared in numerous newspapers, literary journals, and anthologies, including *Best Australian Poems* (2015). Her hybrid memoir (essays/poetry) *Do Oysters Get Bored? A Curious Life* (UWA Publishing) was shortlisted for the National Biography Award in 2019. A chapbook, *The Lady in the Bottle*, is forthcoming from Eyewear (UK).

Kate Lilley (1960–) is a queer, feminist poet-scholar based in Sydney. Her first book, *Versary* (Salt, 2002), won the Grace Leven Prize. Her second, *Ladylike* (UWAP, 2012), was shortlisted for the NSW Premier's Prize. Her most recent book, *Tilt* (Vagabond, 2018), won the Victorian Premier's Award for Poetry in 2019. She is the editor of *Dorothy Hewett: Selected Poems* (UWAP, 2010) and *Margaret Cavendish: The Blazing World and Other Writings* (Penguin Classics).

Nyaluak M Leth – Model/Poet/Actress.

Luka Lesson is a rapper, poet and educator of Greek heritage born in Meanjin / Brisbane. Luka is a former Australian Poetry Slam Champion, has performed with the Queensland Symphony Orchestra, and has his lyrics studied in curricula across the country. Luka has toured with Akala (UK), Lowkey (UK) and Dr Cornel West (USA). He has released two of his own collections of poetry, two full-length albums of musical works, and recently premiered his latest project *Agapi & Other Kinds of Love*, based on Plato's Symposium, at the National Museum of Australia.

Jacinta Le Plastrier is a poet, writer and editor who lives and writes on Boon Wurrung and Wurundjeri Woi Wurrung lands. Her poetry book, inspired by the connectivity between poetic and magical practices, is due early 2023.

Karen Knight has been widely published and anthologised since the early 1960s. She has written four collections of poetry, some of which have won major literary awards, including the 2005 Dorothy Hewett Flagship Fellowship Award and the 2007 Arts ACT Alec Bolton Award. Karen lives on the Tasman Peninsula in a 1910 cottage overlooking Saltwater River with her husband Jules and a menagerie of rescued animals.

Krissy Kneen is the author of the memoir *Affection* and the novels *Steeplechase, Triptych, The Adventures of Holly White and the Incredible Sex Machine* and Stella Prize-shortlisted *An Uncertain Grace*. They are also the author of the Thomas Shapcott Award-winning poetry collection *Eating My Grandmother*. Krissy was the 2020 Copyright Agency Non-fiction Fellow and the resulting book, *Fat Girl Dancing*, will be published in 2023. Krissy has previously written and directed broadcast television documentaries with SBS and ABC TV and is developing a TV series for Stan. Their latest book is the memoir *The Three Burials of Lotty Kneen*.

Paula Keogh is an apprentice poet dedicated to living life as a poem. Her passions are wilderness and nature, poetry, music and stories, and she strives to live with radical hope for the world. She is a writer and the author of *The Green Bell: A Memoir Of Love, Madness And Poetry*, which was shortlisted for the NSW Premier's Award for Non-Fiction and longlisted for the Stella Prize. She has a PhD in Creative Writing and has recently completed a novel. She lives in Melbourne.

Lesh Karan was born in Fiji, has Indian genes and lives in Melbourne. Read her work in *Australian Poetry Journal, Brevity, Cordite Poetry Review, Mascara Literary Review, Island* and *Rabbit*, amongst others. Lesh is undertaking a Master of Creative Writing, Publishing and Editing at the University of Melbourne.

Saanjana Kapoor is a Bachelor of Arts student at the University of Melbourne. Her writing has been published in *Voiceworks*, *Island*, *Cordite Poetry Review* and more. She is the 2022 Writer in Residence at Albert Park College.

Gabrielle Journey Jones is a loud, brown, out and proud poet, percussionist and community builder living on Yuin Country, Far South Coast, New South Wales. Gabrielle has featured her spoken word performances at local, national and international events for twenty-five years. Gabrielle has two poetry collections published by Ginninderra Press, *Etymology of Courage* (2021) and *Spoken Medicine* (2017). Gabrielle has also contributed to a range of exciting Australian anthologies in recent years. She has established many creative projects for individual and community empowerment, three highlights being ongoing initiatives through Creative Womyn Down Under (2006), Poetic Percussion (2018) and Sapphire Coast Pride (2022).

Sandy Jeffs was diagnosed with schizophrenia in 1976 when it was considered something from which you could not recover. In the 1980s, she was among the first wave of people who started speaking publicly about living with a mental illness. Much of her writing has been about her struggle with schizophrenia. Sandy has published eight volumes of poetry and a memoir, *Flying with Paper Wings: Reflections on Living with Madness*. Sandy co-authored with Margaret Leggatt *Out of the Madhouse: From Asylums to Caring Community?* Her most recent publication is *The Poetics of a Plague: A Haiku Diary*.

Anna Jacobson is a poet and artist from Brisbane. *Amnesia Findings* (UQP, 2019) is her first full-length poetry collection, which won the 2018 Thomas Shapcott Poetry Prize. In 2020 Anna won the Nillumbik Prize for Contemporary Writing (Open Creative Nonfiction), was awarded a Queensland Writers Fellowship, and was shortlisted in the Spark Prize. In 2018 she won the Queensland Premier's Young Publishers and Writers Award. Her poetry chapbook *The Last Postman* was published with Vagabond Press (2018) as part of the decibel 3 series. Her website is www.annajacobson.com.au.

KJ lives in Bendigo, Australia, with her wife, their son, three cats and a dog. She writes stories and poems because her imagination takes the wheel. Permanently anxious, a bit mental, and overly fond of her cats, KJ has been told that she's contagiously happy and rather funny. That last one is debatable.

Holly Isemonger is the author of the chapbooks *Hip Shifts* (If A Leaf Falls Press) and *Deluxe Paperweight* (Stale Objects dePress). She can be found at @Hisemonger on Twitter.

Martin Ingle is a writer, filmmaker and obsessive-compulsive worrywart who works on Yuggera land. His comedy-drama script *Disorderly* is in development and was an international finalist for the prestigious ScreenCraft Fellowship. He is also a fierce advocate, featuring in the OCD episode of the ABC's *You Can't Ask That* and in comedy series about OCD, *Plushed*, currently in development with Screen Australia. He's one of five contributors to OCD anthology *Try Not To Think Of A Pink Elephant* with Fremantle Press, and his writing has been published in *The Guardian*, *ABC News Online*, *The Chaser* and *The Shovel*.

Darby Hudson is a writer and artist from Melbourne, Australia, previously included in *Best Australian Poems* (Black Inc. Book, 2012 and 2013).

Ruby Hillsmith is a writer, editor and poet based in Melbourne, on Wurundjeri land. She was the 2020 Writeability poetry fellow at Writers Victoria and a 2020–21 Wheeler Centre Hot Desk Fellow. She aims to produce work that is the poetic equivalent of the smiling imp emoji.

Tim Heffernan has published at *Thylazine*, *Cordite*, *Spineless Wonders*, *Eureka Street*, *Blackmail Press*, *Red Room Poetry* and *Verity La*. Most recently his work has appeared in *Australian Poetry*, *Rabbit* and *Plumwood Mountain*. Tim was awarded the 2016 joanne burns Award for prose poetry and microfiction. With poet Alise Blayney he developed the first MAD Poetry' workshops and readings at the

2016 Wollongong Writers Festival and together they co-edit *Verity La*'s 'Clozapine Clinic – The Frater Project'. Tim has also collaborated with Iraqi poet Haider Catan in translating 'Poetry in the Minefield', published in *Verity La*'s 'Discoursing Diaspora'.

Jenny Hedley writes about mental illness and domestic abuse from a position of lived experience. She's looking for a publisher for her fictocritical memoir on gendered violence and is writing speculatively on her mother's inaccessible archives. She lives on unceded Boon Wurrung land with her son. Jennyhedley.github.io

Justin Heazlewood is the author of *Funemployed: Life as an Artist in Australia* (2014). 'Thinking is drilling' is taken from his 2018 childhood memoir, *Get Up Mum*, about living with a mum with schizophrenia. In 2020 he gave a witness statement for the Royal Commission into Victoria's Mental Health System. He is an ambassador for Satellite Foundation, which supports young people caring for a mentally ill parent. He is set to act his life out in a one-man theatre adaptation of *Get Up Mum* in 2022 and beyond. www.justinheazlewood.com

Amani Haydar is an award-winning writer, visual artist, lawyer and advocate for women's health and safety based in Western Sydney. Amani's debut memoir, *The Mother Wound* (Pan Macmillan), was awarded the 2022 Victorian Premier's Literary Award for Non-fiction. Amani's writing and illustrations have featured in several publications, including *Arab Australian Other*, *Sweatshop Women Volume Two*, *Racism*, *SBS Voices* and *ABC News Online*.

Olivia Hamilton writes poetry and speculative fiction that explores the experiences of chronic pain, mental illness and neurodivergence as well as the intersections between the intimacies of everyday life and big issues like climate change and inequality. She lives in Newcastle, New South Wales, with her husband and dog.

Lajos Hamers is a storyteller of Hungarian folk tales, actor, writer, musician and survivor. He hails from Canberra but now calls Wollongong home. Here he is active in the creative community and volunteers for a local AFL sports team, the University of Wollongong Bulldogs.

Rachael Wenona Guy is a multifaceted artist in theatre, puppetry and visual art as well as a published author. She holds a BFA, Postgraduate Diploma in Puppetry and a Master's in Theatre Production. She is fascinated by themes of ambivalence, bodily experience and identity. In recent years she has collaborated with poet Andy Jackson on poetry/puppetry theatre works *Ambiguous Mirrors* and *Each Map of Scars*. Her stop-motion puppet animation *Secessionist* with Leonie Van Eyk and Andy won an outstanding achievement award at the Berlin Flash Film Festival 2017. Rachael's writing has appeared in numerous journals, including *Sleepers Almanac*, *Overland* and *Australian Poetry Journal*. In 2020 Rachael published her debut poetry collection, *The Hungry Air*, with Walleah Press.

Maddie Godfrey is a writer, educator and emotional feminist. They have performed their poetry at the Sydney Opera House, St Paul's Cathedral and Glastonbury Festival (2017). Maddie is a previous recipient of the Kat Muscat Fellowship and the Varuna Poetry Flagship Fellowship, and was recently awarded a Western Australian Youth Award for their 'Creative Contributions' to the state. Their debut collection, *How To Be Held* (Burning Eye Books, 2018), is a manifesto to tenderness. Maddie is completing their PhD and living on Whadjuk Noongar land with a rescue cat named Sylvia.

Andrew Galan works on Ngunnawal Country. Published in Australia and internationally, he performs at events and festivals regularly. His book, *For All The Veronicas (The Dog Who Staid)*, Bareknuckle Books, won an ACT Writing and Publishing Award. He co-edited *Australian Poetry Journal*'s first volume of spoken word and performance poetry, 8.2 – 'spoken', and has produced and curated events for over ten years. He most recently worked with Southern Tablelands Arts as a mentor and commissioned poet, has work forthcoming in anthologies, was an inaugural member of the Australian Capital Territory Arts Minister's Creative Council.

Alan Fyfe is a Jewish writer living on Whajuk Noongar Boodjar. His poetry largely uses philosophy and non-poetry referents for its material and concerns. Alan's first novel, *T*, was shortlisted for Australian and international awards, and is now available from Transit Lounge Press.

Benjamin Frater (1979–2007) was raised in Sydney's Campbelltown area, attending Airds High School and later the University of Wollongong. There, calling himself and known to many as 'The Catholic Yak', he needed to cope with his emerging schizophrenia. Heading an energetic group of fellow poets, he became the university's unofficial Poet-in-Residence. If enamoured with and earlier influenced by Allen Ginsberg, his tastes and works extended well beyond those of the Beats. Benjamin's death being a big loss for our poetry, his *6am in the Universe: Selected Poems* was published in 2011.

Helena Fox lives on Dharawal Country, in Wollongong, Australia, where she mentors young writers and runs workshops on writing and mental health. Her debut novel, *How It Feels to Float*, published in Australia and internationally, won the Prime Minister's Literary Award and Victorian Premier's Literary Award for Writing for Young Adults. Helena received her MFA in Creative Writing from Warren Wilson College in the USA.

Ela Fornalska has performed her work nationally and internationally, at festivals, on television, the radio, and a tram. She has been published in journals and anthologies and was shortlisted in Red Room Poetry's 'Poetry Object' competition and won Wordcraft Spoken Word slam. *The Dance Inside* is her first full-length collection.

Es Foong is a poet living in Naarm (Melbourne). She wants you to know that you are a wild, precious and unique expression of possibility and you are cherished. Onstage, she is the poetic analogue of heavy-metal karaoke. Offstage, she is having an identity crisis. She lives online at www.waffleirongirl.com.

Chris Fleming is a writer and translator whose work has appeared in the scholarly and popular media, including, mostly recently, *Westerly*, *The Guardian*, *The Saturday Paper*, *The LA Review of Books* and *The Chronicle Review*. He is the author or editor of ten books, including *Modern Conspiracy: The Importance of Being Paranoid* (Bloomsbury, 2014) and *On Drugs* (Giramondo, 2019). He is Associate Professor in Humanities and a Member of the Writing and Society Research Centre at Western Sydney University.

Michael Farrell grew up in Bombala, New South Wales, and has lived in Melbourne since 1990. Recent books include *Family Trees, I Love Poetry* (both Giramondo) and the edited anthology *Ashbery Mode* (TinFish). The poem and artwork featured in this anthology derive largely from experiences of 2020–21, including clinic stays. Michael's artwork can be found on instagram @limechax.

Heidi Everett is a writer, award-winning multidisciplinary artist, independent producer, mental health creative recovery advocate and neurodiversity consultant based in Melbourne / on Wurundjeri Country. As the Founder and Director of Schizy Inc, Mojo Film Festival and Qualia Theatre, Heidi enables people with diverse mental health experiences to engage with the arts as storytellers and contributors. Heidi's memoir, *My Friend Fox*, is widely available, published by Ultimo Press.

Gabrielle Everall has a PhD in Creative Writing. The second edition of her book *Dona Juanita and the love of boys* was published with Buon-Cattivi Press. John Kinsella included *Dona Juanita and the love of boys* as one of the best poetry books for 2020 in *Australian Book Review*. She has been published in numerous anthologies including *The Penguin Anthology of Australian Poetry*. She has performed her poetry at La Mama, The Bowery in New York and the Edinburgh Fringe Festival. She has also performed her work at the Evil Women conference in Vienna.

Ali Cobby Eckermann is a Yankunytjatjara poet whose first collection, *little bit long time*, was written in the desert in 2009. Ali has been blessed by her writings receiving much recognition. Ali is the first Aboriginal Australian writer to attend the International Writing Program in Iowa in 2014, and in 2017 Ali received a Windham Campbell Prize for Poetry from Yale University, USA.

Quinn Eades is a Senior Lecturer in Gender, Sexuality and Diversity Studies at La Trobe University, Melbourne. A writer, researcher, editor and poet, his book *Rallying* was awarded the 2018 Mary Gilmore Award for best first book of poetry. He is the author of *all the beginnings: a queer autobiography of the body* and is currently writing two books: *is the body home*, an autobiography from the transitioning body; and an essay collection titled *Collaboration as Love*. Quinn's practice-led research is grounded in experimental and hybrid writing practices and works across/through trans, queer, and feminist theories of the body, poetry and life writing.

Kristen Dunphy has thirty years experience writing, creating and producing drama for Australian television. She has received numerous awards for screenwriting on shows such as *The Straits*, *Eastwest 101* and *White Collar Blue*. In 2012 she was awarded the Foxtel Fellowship in recognition of the significant contribution she has made to Australian screenwriting. In 2014 she co-created and co-wrote *The Principal* and in 2021 she created, co-wrote and produced *Wakefield*, an eight x one-hour miniseries for Jungle Entertainment, the ABC and BBC Studios. The series screened on Showtime in the USA in October 2021.

Jonathan Dunk is the co-editor of *Overland* and a Lecturer in Writing and Literature at Deakin University. He lives on Wurundjeri country.

Shastra Deo was born in Fiji, raised in Melbourne and lives in Brisbane. Her first book, *The Agonist* (UQP 2017), won the 2016 Arts Queensland Thomas Shapcott Poetry Prize and the 2018 Australian Literature Society Gold Medal. Her second book, *The Exclusion Zone*, is forthcoming from University of Queensland Press in 2023.

Kristen de Kline writes poetry by night and lectures in Criminology by day. Their poetry appears in different publications, including *Backstory, Other Terrain, Pink Cover Zine, Burrow, Guide to Sydney Crime, Australian Poetry Collaboration, Press: 100 Love Letters* and *Project 365+1*. Kristen's debut collection, *Lawless*, was published by Girls on Key in 2021.

Kobie Dee is a 24-year-old Gomeroi artist from Maroubra in South Sydney, Bidjigal Land. With an innate gift for storytelling and connecting with young people, Kobie Dee is one of the exciting new voices in Australian hip-hop. Kobie was signed to Bad Apples Music in 2019 and has performed alongside artists including Briggs, Jessica Mauboy, Nooky and Barkaa as part of Yabun, Sydney Festival, and at the Bad Apples House Party at the Sydney Opera House. In 2019 Kobie performed as the support act for UK artist Dave as part of his Psychodrama Tour at the Enmore Theatre. As an artist, Kobie is deeply engaged in his community through performance and community work, and his passion for his culture and people is inspiring new generations. Kobie is passionate about advocating for systemic change to help reduce the overrepresentation of Aboriginal young people in custody and improving mental health access for young people, and has shared his lived experience of navigating life's challenges to numerous audiences around Australia.

Josie/Jocelyn Deane is a programmer/translator. They are one of the recipients of the 2021 Next Chapter Fellowship. They are a genderqueer trans femme. They live on unceded Wurundjeri land in Naarm.

Aloma Davis is an emerging poet whose works feature a direct and intimate voice. She invites readers to question their worldview by exploring the everyday things in life we take for granted. Based in Melbourne, Australia, she collects bad jokes and good fluffy cats.

Andrew Cox is a proud Filipino/Australian who creates and lives on Ngunnawal & Ngambri Country (Canberra) Australia. Currently, Andrew produces and leads Canberra Poetry Slam, the capital's new and exciting home for stories and spoken word. Andrew's work has been shortlisted for national writing prizes, notably for the Emily XYZ prize for Innovation in Spoken Word and his writing published in multiple anthologies.

Radhiah Chowdhury is an author, audio producer and editor living on unceded Bidjigal Land in Sydney's south-west. Together with Camha Pham and Grace Lucas-Pennington, she is one of the founders and moderators of the Australian First Nations and People of Colour in Publishing Network, and was the 2019–2020 Beatrice Davis Editorial Fellow, awarded for her research paper, 'It's hard to be what you can't see: Diversity Within Australian Publishing'. As an editor, Radhiah has worked with Scholastic Australia, Giramondo, Allen & Unwin and Penguin Random House. Her most recent picture book, *The Katha Chest* (Allen & Unwin, 2021), is a 2022 CBCA Notable for Picture Book of the Year.

Jen Chen is an Australian Chinese poet and lawyer (@jen.chen. rhymes). She has worked in international aid, domestic violence policy and mental health law. Her work has been published by *Verity La*, SBS, Hunter Writers Centre and Manly Art Gallery and Museum. Her work explores themes of justice, resilience and family.

Wendy Burton is living independently in the place of her dreams.

Pascalle Burton is an experimental writer based in Meanjin. Her collection *About the Author is Dead* is available from Cordite Books. She also plays in the band The Stress of Leisure.

John Mukky Burke lives in Wagga Wagga and was born in Narrandera in 1946. His mother was the daughter of a resident of Warangesda Mission at Darlington Point, New South Wales, and his father was of Irish heritage. Because of his fair skin, identification as Wiradjuri has been a longtime battle. Because of his position on the sexual spectrum, he likewise has taken ages to be comfortable with what is basically not a clearly binary situation. Both ethnicity and sexuality are arguably among the most fraught dimensions humans have to deal with. Mukky's latest collection is *Late Murrumbidgee Poems* (Cordite, 2020).

Jean Burke returned to writing poetry when burnt out from academic work. She now works as a Swahili translator, having learnt this language when living in Tanzania. Writing helps Jean experience wellbeing and meaning while managing the chronic pain and fatigue of fibromyalgia and its cognitive and mental health challenges.

Together with her entourage of diagnoses, **Rosie Bogumil** writes unapologetically about mental illness. She is fascinated by the interplay between page and stage – so much so that it became a dissertation. Rosie has previously received the Randolph Stow Young Writers Award six consecutive times, and her first collection of poetry, *Decorating Pain*, was published in 2021.

Alise Blayney is a poet and peer educator with extensive experience in peer work and recovery-focused education across mental health settings.

Currently working on Gadigal Land, **Sophie Bellotti**'s multi-disciplinary practice explores the interplay of matter and language, and how language carves and becomes material reality in socially and culturally situated ways. She holds a Bachelor of Arts (Honours) in Creative Writing and Linguistics from the University of Melbourne.

Ethan Bell is a Wallabalooa man from the Ngunawal Nation. He is an emerging artist and writer based in Campbelltown, Sydney. Ethan's practice involves storytelling, production and education. Ethan writes poetry to give insight into his life. His work has been published by *Red Room Poetry*, Magabala Books and Sydney Living Museums. He is an artist educator at the Museum of Contemporary Art in Sydney and is studying a Bachelor of Arts at Western Sydney University.

The Bedroom Philosopher discovered irony from a mail-in voucher on the back of a *That's Life* magazine. He quickly taught himself music on a Melody Pop and a guitar he built in grade eight woodwork.

His first song was about *Home & Away* and his second song was about depression. He is currently a success and his albums fetch lira on Pinterest. www.bedroomphilosopher.com

Stuart Barnes is the author of two poetry collections: *Like To The Lark* (Upswell Publishing, 2023) and *Glasshouses* (UQP, 2016), which won the 2015 Arts Queensland Thomas Shapcott Prize, was commended for the 2016 Anne Elder Award, and was shortlisted for the 2017 Mary Gilmore Award. 'Sestina after B. Carlisle' won the 2021/22 Gwen Harwood Poetry Prize. Recently he guest-edited, with Claire Gaskin, *Australian Poetry Journal 11.1 – 'local, attention'*. He tweets and grams as @StuartABarnes. Stuartabarnes.com

Spencer Barberis is undertaking Honours in Creative Writing at University of Wollongong with a focus on lyrical poetry and hybrid forms. He is a co-founder of the forthcoming journal *Bramble*. Spencer splits his time between Wiradjuri and Dharawal lands.

Mary Baker grew up alongside her two brothers, Jack and Henri, in a loving home. The youngest of the three, she was an avid horserider, swimmer and water polo player. In 2011 Mary took her life, aged just fifteen years. Her tragic death came after she was diagnosed with an eating disorder three years earlier. Mary loved poetry and connected strongly to the works of Shaun Tan, in particular *The Red Tree*, an illustrated story about a girl struggling to find hope and her place in a dark, confusing world.

After losing their beloved daughter, Mary, to suicide in 2011, **Annette and Stuart Baker** have become leaders in their community in breaking down barriers surrounding suicide and mental illness. In the days following Mary's death the couple came across two poems she had written for a school assignment, which also included an anthology on several poems that Mary had chosen. Mary's raw and devastating words gave Stuart and Annette a glimpse into the suffering and despair she had endured at the hands of an eating disorder and her poems continue to inspire their work today.

Mohammad Awad is a Queer/Arab/Muslim and Writer/Director/Poet/Playwright who's running out of ways to express himself. He has written and directed short films such as The Flower, The Messenger and Beauty Marks. Published in an anthology series 'Arab, Australian, Other' as well as The University of Sydney Student Anthology 'Diversity', he is also one of the proud editors of this anthology collection *Admissions*. He has featured in every iconic West Ball, as well as in the Sydney Writers Festival, Sydney Mardi Gras, Sydney Living Museums – After Dark, The ICC, Sydney Festival, Word in Hand, Red Room Poetry, Giant Dwarf Theatre.

Evelyn Araluen is a poet, researcher and co-editor of *Overland*. Her widely published criticism, fiction and poetry has been awarded the Nakata Brophy Prize for Young Indigenous Writers, the Judith Wright Poetry Prize, a Wheeler Centre Next Chapter Fellowship and a Neilma Sidney Literary Travel Fund grant. Born and raised on Dharug country, she is a descendant of the Bundjalung Nation. Evelyn's debut collection, *Dropbear*, was shortlisted for the 2021 Judith Wright Calanthe Award for a Poetry Collection and won the 2022 Stella Prize.

Christine Anu is one of Australia's most popular recording artists and performers of all time. With seventeen ARIA nominations, including the APRA AMCOS award-winning 'My Island Home' and her platinum album *Stylin' Up*, she has one of the country's most enduring and recognisable voices. Her acclaimed 27-year career spans across all forms of media, including music, theatre, dance, film, television, radio and children's entertainment. Christine is and will always be proud of her Torres Strait Islander heritage and at any given opportunity will use her public profile as a platform to advocate for Aboriginal and Torres Strait Islander people.

Eunice Andrada is a poet and educator. Her first poetry collection, *Flood Damages* (Giramondo Publishing, 2018), won the Anne Elder Award and was shortlisted for the Victorian Premier's Literary Award for Poetry and the Dame Mary Gilmore Award. *TAKE CARE* is her second poetry collection. Born and raised in the Philippines, she lives and writes on unceded Gadigal Land.

Steph Amir has a background in research, including in public health, and was a Writers Victoria Writeability Fellow in 2021. Her poems have been published online and in print internationally, and in Australian publications such as *Baby Teeth Journal*, *Burrow*, *Echidna Tracks*, *Mantissa Poetry Review* and *The Victorian Writer*. She lives in Melbourne.

Maja Amanita is a poet and writer based in Cairns. She has been published in *Meanjin* and *Antithesis*, has contributed playwriting for Theatreworks production *She is Vigilante*, and is writing her first full-length play for theatre.

Dr **Claire Albrecht** is a poet, editor and curator from Mulubinba (Newcastle), New South Wales. She was the 2019 Emerging Writers Festival fellow at the State Library of Victoria, a 2020 Varuna 'Writing Fire, Writing Drought' fellow and the 2021 West Darling Arts Writer in Residence. She will (Covid willing) be a resident at the Helene Wurlitzer Foundation, New Mexico, in 2022. Claire's debut chapbook, *pinky swear*, was published in 2018, and her book *handshake* was shortlisted for the Puncher & Wattmann First Poetry Book Prize.

Acknowledgements

Works from this collection have appeared previously in the following books and journals, some as earlier versions:

Ellen van Neerven's **Memories sometimes come backwards** first appeared in *Throat*, UQP, 2020

Sam Twyford-Moore's **Preface to *The Rapids*** first appeared as the Preface to *The Rapids*, University of Toronto Press, 2020

Elizabeth Tan's **Smart Ovens for Lonely People** first appeared in *Smart Ovens for Lonely People*, Brio Books, 2020

Grace Tame's **Hard Pressed** first appeared on *Red Room Poetry* commissioned as part of Poetry Month, 2021

David Stavanger's **Suicide Dogs** first appeared on *Red Room Poetry*, 2020; also appears in *Case Notes*, UWAP, 2020

Kirli Saunders' **Wallflowers and Evergreens** first appeared in *Returning*, Magabala Books, 2023; and in a film by Tad Souden.

Rebecca Rushbrook's **The Queue** first appeared on *Red Room Poetry* commissioned as part of MAD Poetry, 2020

Anne Ross' **At the psychiatrist's office seeking hormones like a thirsty snail seeking water, soft and gooey but hiding my insides** first appeared on *#EnbyLife*, 2020

Lillian Rodrigues-Pang's **Permission to forget** first appeared on *Red Room Poetry* commissioned as part of MAD Poetry, 2020

Steven Oliver's **CARRY ALL MY HURT AWAY** appears in his comedy-cabaret show *Bigger & Blacker*

Omar Musa's **Paleochannel** first appeared in *Killernova*, Penguin, 2021

Scott-Patrick Mitchell's **my body is a window** first appeared on *Red Room Poetry* commissioned as part of MAD Poetry, 2021

Misha the maniac's **Septic tank universe** first appeared on *Red Room Poetry* commissioned as part of MAD Poetry, 2020; also appears in *Ivris*, Apothecary Press, 2021

Anthony Mannix's **Intricately and Intimately Fractured** first appeared on *Red Room Poetry* commissioned as part of MAD Poetry, 2020

Luka Lesson's **Bones** first appeared in *Antidote*, 2015

Karen Knight's **Renovating Madness** first appeared in *Renovating Madness*, Walleah Press, 2018

Gabrielle Journey Jones' **Triptych: Post Traumatic Relationship Syndrome** first appeared on *Red Room Poetry* commissioned as part of MAD Poetry, 2021

Sandy Jeffs' **The Madwoman in this Poem** first appeared in *The Mad Poet's Tea Party*, Spinifex Press, 2015

Holly Isemonger and Chris Fleming's **Comic Sans** first appeared on *Red Room Poetry* commissioned as part of MAD Poetry, 2020

An earlier version of Martin Ingle's **A victim who feels like a villain** appeared on *ABC Online*, 2021

Darby Hudson's **100 Points of ID to Prove I Don't Exist** first appeared in *Falling Upwards*, Five Islands Press, 2019

Tim Heffernan's **from the book of puns and other altered sentences** first appeared on *Red Room Poetry* commissioned as part of MAD Poetry, 2020

Justin Heazlewood's **Thinking is drilling** first appeared in *Get Up Mum*, Affirm Press, 2018

Benjamin Frater's **The Argument** first appeared in *6am in the Universe*, Grande Parade Poets, 2011

Helena Fox's **dissociate is to** first appeared on *Red Room Poetry* commissioned as part of MAD Poetry, 2020

Gabrielle Everall's **Pear of Anguish** first appeared in *Rabbit*, Issue 27 – Tense, 2019

Jonathan Dunk's **Ghost Song** first appeared on *Red Room Poetry* commissioned as part of MAD Poetry, 2020

Kobie Dee's **Role Models** first appeared on *Red Room Poetry* commissioned as part of MAD Poetry, 2020

John Mukky Burke's **ON WAKING UP IN THE WARD AT OAKLEY** first appeared in *Night Song and Other Poems*, NTU Press, 1999

John Mukky Burke's **Medical Nemesis** first appeared in *Late Murrumbidgee Poems*, Cordite, 2020

Alise Blayney's **The Z–A of Crazy** first appeared on *Red Room Poetry* commissioned as part of MAD Poetry, 2020

The Bedroom Philosopher's **I'm So Lonely** first appeared on the album *Brown and Orange*, 2009

Stuart Barnes' **Sestina: Rape** first appeared in *The Moth*, Autumn Issue, 2020

Mary Baker's **The Key** and Annette and Stuart Baker's **Reflections on 'The Key'** first appeared on *Red Room Poetry* commissioned as part of MAD Poetry, 2021

Evelyn Araluen's **Interior Anxious** was first commissioned by *The Big Anxiety* as a video-poem, 2019

Christine Anu's **Better Out Than In** first appeared on *Red Room Poetry* commissioned as part of MAD Poetry, 2020

Eunice Andrada's **Sexual Assault Report Questionnaire: Describe your hair.** first appeared in *TAKE CARE*, Giramondo, 2021

Claire Albrecht's **Annexiety** first appeared in *Overland*, Issue 231, 2018

Supporters

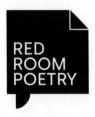

Red Room Poetry (RR) is Australia's leading organisation for creating, commissioning, publishing and promoting poetry in meaningful ways. RR's support of MAD Poetry, since giving it a home as a core project in 2020, has led to lived experience poets across Australia being commissioned – and paid – to write about their mental health and illness on their own terms. Half the pieces within this book have come about via RR's direct involvement, including the thirty emerging voices selected for this anthology as part of their open call-out.

We thank RR for being a key anthology partner and lived experience supporter. Special thanks to Anne-Marie Te Whiu, who was a previous MAD Poetry workshop facilitator and part of an early iteration of *Admissions* as it first took shape, as well as Dr Tamryn Bennett, who has unreservedly backed this initiative and the need to create safe creative spaces for marginalised voices to reclaim language and express how they see the world.

For more information on the MAD Poetry project:
redroompoetry.org/projects/mad-poetry

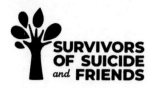

Survivors of Suicide & Friends (SOSF) was formed around loss.
Annette and Stuart Baker, co-founders of SOSF, lost their daughter
Mary to suicide in 2011. Not only have they come on board as a
project partner to support some of the commissions in *Admissions*,
they have also agreed to have one of Mary's poems and their own
personal reflections on her writing and life included within these
pages. We thank them for their broader work in this space, their
warm hearts, and the way they open up conversations that too few of
us are willing to have.

For more information on SOSF: https://survivorsofsuicide.org.au

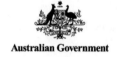 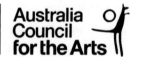

This project has been assisted by the Australian Government through
the Australia Council, its arts funding and advisory body.

And last but far from least, huge thanks to Alex Adsett for truly advocating for and taking on *Admissions* and to Upswell Publishing, in particular Terri-ann, for backing this project on its own terms and giving these voices a print home. Deepest gratitude from the editorial team.

About Upswell

Upswell Publishing was established in
2021 by Terri-ann White as a not-for-profit
press. A perceived gap in the market for
distinctive literary works in fiction, poetry
and narrative non-fiction was the motivation.
In her years as a bookseller, writer and then
publisher, Terri-ann has maintained a watch
on literary books and the way they insinuate
themselves into a cultural space and are
then located within our literary and cultural
inheritance. She is interested in making books
to last: books with the potential to still be
noticed, and noted, after decades and thus
be ripe to influence new literary histories.

About this typeface

Book designer Becky Chilcott chose
Foundry Origin not only as a strong,
carefully considered, and dependable
typeface, but also to honour her late
friend and mentor, type designer Freda
Sack, who oversaw the project. Designed
by Freda's long-standing colleague,
Stuart de Rozario, much like Upswell
Publishing, Foundry Origin was created
out of the desire to say something new.